Easy Gourmet
Baby Food

Easy Gourmet Baby Food

150 Recipes for Homemade Goodness

Chef Jordan Wagman & Jill Hillhouse, BPHE, RNCP

Robert ROSE

Easy Gourmet Baby Food
Text copyright © 2008 Jordan Wagman and Jill Hillhouse
Color Food Photographs copyright © 2008 Robert Rose Inc.
Cover and text design copyright © 2008 Robert Rose Inc.

For complete cataloguing information, see page 244.

Disclaimer

The recipes in this book have been carefully tested by our kitchen and our tasters. To the best of our knowledge, they are safe and nutritious for ordinary use and users. For those people with food or other allergies, or who have special food requirements or health issues, please read the suggested contents of each recipe carefully and determine whether or not they may create a problem for you. All recipes are used at the risk of the consumer.

We cannot be responsible for any hazards, loss or damage that may occur as a result of any recipe use.

For those with special needs, allergies, requirements or health problems, in the event of any doubt, please contact your medical adviser prior to the use of any recipe.

Design and Production: Kevin Cockburn/PageWave Graphics Inc.
Editor: Judith Finlayson
Copy Editor: Karen Campbell-Sheviak
Proofreaders: Karen Campbell-Sheviak and Gillian Watts
Recipe Tester: Jennifer MacKenzie
Indexer: Gillian Watts

Interior Color Photography (Food): Colin Erricson
Food Styling: Kathryn Robertson
Prop Styling: Charlene Erricson

Interior Color Photography (Babies): © Masterfile (opposite page 64),
© Vivid Pixels, 2008. Used under license from Shutterstock.com (opposite page 65),
© SaferTim, 2008. Used under license from Shutterstock.com (opposite page 96),
© Magdalena Szachowska, 2008. Used under license from Shutterstock.com (opposite page 97),
© 2008 Jupiterimages Corporation (opposite page 160),
© iStockphoto.com/Ieva Geneviciene (opposite page 161),
© Brooke Fasani/Corbis (opposite page 192),
© iStockphoto.com/Lara Seregni (opposite page 193)

Interior Black & White Photography: © iStockphoto.com/Ashok Rodrigues (page 9),
© iStockphoto.com/Zoran Mircetic (page 13), © iStockphoto.com/Andrey Shchekalev (page 29),
© iStockphoto.com/Kamel Adjenef (page 30), © iStockphoto.com/Petr Nad (page 78),
© iStockphoto.com/Jelani Memory (page 112), © iStockphoto.com/Pauline Vos (page 168),
© iStockphoto.com/Christoph Ermel (page 198)

Cover image: © Norbert Schäfer/Masterfile

We acknowledge the financial support of the Government of Canada through the Book Publishing Industry Development Program (BPIDP) for our publishing activities.

Published by Robert Rose Inc.
120 Eglinton Avenue East, Suite 800, Toronto, Ontario, Canada M4P 1E2
Tel: (416) 322-6552 Fax: (416) 322-6936

Printed and bound in Canada
1 2 3 4 5 6 7 8 9 CPL 16 15 14 13 12 11 10 09 08

Contents

Acknowledgments 6

Nutrient Analysis 8

From the Chef 10

From the Nutritionist 14

Preparing Your Own Baby Food 26

∎ ∎ ∎

Starting Solids (6 to 9 Months) 31

Establishing Preferences (9 to 12 Months) 79

Food for Toddlers (12 Months +) 113

Snacks and Desserts 169

Not for Adults Only 199

∎ ∎ ∎

Index 245

Acknowledgments

Looking back at my culinary career, it's difficult to remember and thank every teacher, line cook, dishwasher or manager who has influenced my career. But there are a few who have been instrumental in my professional and personal growth and I've waited a long time to formally thank them.

To my culinary mentors, Chef Oliver Saucy, Chef Gianni Respinto, Chef Doug Zuk, Chef Mark McEwen, Chef Brad Long and Chef Pascal Olhats: In one way or another, you have instilled in me a superb work ethic and inherent need for being the best at my craft by simply loving what I do — cook. I am indebted to you all.

More recently, thank you to Sweetpea Baby Food for the springboard to opportunity. To Robert Rose Publishing, specifically Bob Dees, thank you for granting me this tremendous learning experience. To Michael Levine, thank you.

To the family at Cuisinart, thank you for providing me with the greatest kitchen equipment to test hundreds of recipes. There is no substitute for good quality and yours is simply the best.

To my very close friends, whom I consider family, thank you.

To my family, who are my best friends, I love you. To Mom and Dad, Michelle and Adam, Ryan and Jennifer. To Lee and Hessie, Steve and Mya and all my nieces and nephews: Hayley, Sydney, Josh, Shane and Eryn.

To my two beautiful children, Jonah Max and Jamie Rimon, I truly now know the meaning of life: it's you. I love you. Lastly, where would I be without my muse, my pillar of strength, my sparring partner, travel partner and life partner, Tamar? Probably nowhere! I love you more today than that first day I saw you at summer camp all those years ago. You've stood by me while working 15-hour days in kitchens from Israel to Colorado, every step of the way. My successes have been your own. I look forward to the rest of our life together.

— Jordan Wagman

I'd like to thank my co-author Chef Jordan Wagman for asking me to contribute to this book. Helping parents start their children off with the best possible nutrition is close to my heart and I am delighted to have been a part of this book.

Many thanks to those at PageWave Graphics who have worked on the design and styling of this book, especially Kevin Cockburn. I'd also like to thank copy editor Karen Campbell-Sheviak, recipe editor and tester Jennifer MacKenzie, photographer Colin Erricson, prop stylist Charlene Erricson, food stylist Kathryn Robertson and Marian Jarkovich at Robert Rose for her marketing expertise.

Special thanks to Judith Finlayson for her gentle editorial guidance and Bob Dees at Robert Rose for his vision and commitment to bringing this book to market.

Thanks also to Joey Shulman for her ongoing support and Julia Rickert for her assistance and friendship.

Many thanks to Dr. Piché and Kim Zammit for their work on the nutrient analyses and for their patience as we tweaked recipes.

A final thank you to my parents for starting me on the right nutritional path; to Stewart and Duncan for always agreeing to eat anything I put in front of them and finally to Bob for his constant and profound support.

— Jill Hillhouse

Nutrient Analysis

The nutrient analyses for the recipes in this book were prepared by Kimberly Zammit in conjunction with Professor Leonard Piché, PhD, RD, both of Brescia University College, the University of Western Ontario, London, ON. The analyses were performed with the Food Processor SQL version 10.1, ESHA Research, Inc. Salem, OR.

The nutrient analyses were based on

- imperial measures and weights
- the first ingredient listed when there was a choice
- the exclusion of "optional" ingredients
- the exclusion of ingredients with "non-specified" or "to taste" amounts.

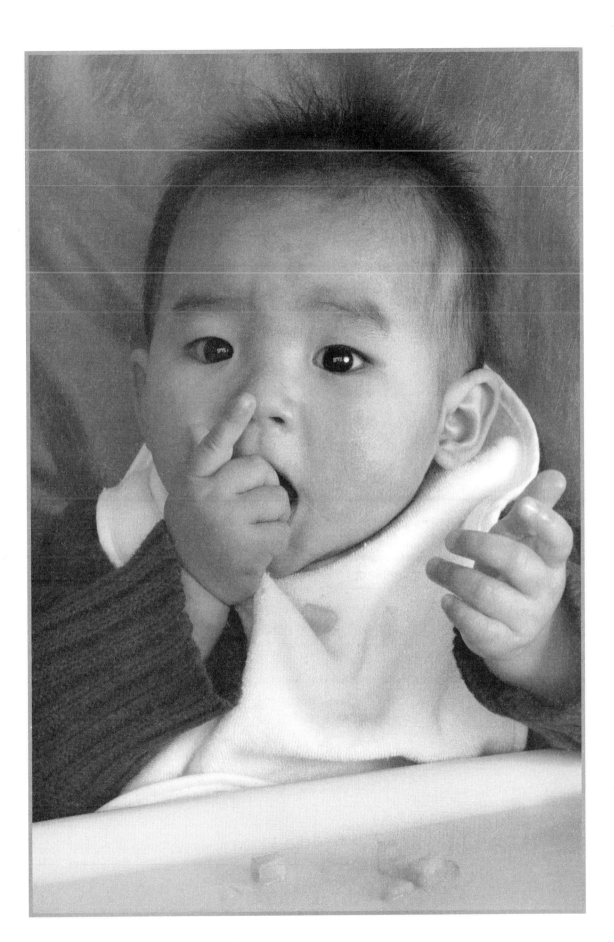

From the Chef

As the only chef in my extended family, I have learned to expect two things. The first is people who randomly drop in right around dinnertime.

"Hey Jord, just came over to drop off...ooooh, what's for dinner?" My family is great, but they're hardly subtle.

The second is recipe requests. Weeks or months after a particular meal, people will call wanting to know how to make a dish they enjoyed. It's not as hard as it may seem to make great gourmet-inspired foods for your family. In fact, I can tell you how to do it in three words: Ingredients. Ingredients. Ingredients.

It may not be breaking news, but it happens to be true. Most chefs will tell you, to cook great food start with the best ingredients, locally grown whenever possible, and manipulate them as little as it takes. Great ingredients make the best meals.

This philosophy is one I've always abided by, particularly in my role as the executive chef of one of the leading frozen organic baby food companies in North America. Kids have educated palates and they can be notoriously harsh critics. If we can tell the difference between a tomato picked fresh from the vine and a tomato grown in South America and allowed to ripen en route to North America, we should assume our children can, too. So in developing the recipes for this book, I chose a very important coauthor — my three-year-old son, executive-chef-in-training, Jonah.

My approach to cooking for Jonah is to create meals based on the ingredients we have on hand, with a basic respect for seasonality and a few simple cooking methods. I also like to be efficient. So when I'm making something for him I prefer to incorporate it into the family meal as well. This strategy has worked very well for my wife and me, even though it may have contributed to Jonah's habit of eating off our plates.

Another technique that has served us well is one my wife, who has no professional training, taught me. Tamar varies the meals that she makes. Unlike my mother (no offense, Mom) she doesn't serve the same dish over and over again. Most people get used to making the same five or six things and never stray too far away from them. This book will help you to break those habits. You'll see possibilities where you used to see, well, a banana.

Tamar also taught me about "changing it up." By that I mean varying the cooking methods for the same ingredients to achieve a different flavor profile. For instance, if your child doesn't like steamed sweet potato, why serve it? Try roasting sweet potato instead, which develops the sugars. Have you ever grilled a peach or roasted a banana? It creates very different flavors.

It's amazing what happens to fruits and vegetables when they are transformed through dry heat. By roasting, you can transform an acorn squash into a piece of candy and watch your kids beg for more. You read that right: My son begs us for more acorn squash. A vegetable. And why? Because we change the cooking methods to trick Jonah into thinking it's a different food when all along, it's the same vegetable he didn't enjoy steamed. We try different things.

When Jonah turned seven months old, we were so excited because we could introduce him to new foods. We began with basic purées and progressed quickly to puréed chicken and beef recipes. It didn't take long to notice that if Jonah didn't like an ingredient (peeled and steamed butternut squash comes to mind), he would refuse to eat it. But if we changed up the cooking method (steamed vs. roasted) just a little — for example, if we roasted the squash whole with the skin still on — he would love it. The reason was obvious — sugar! So many of the fruits and vegetables we eat are full of healthy, natural sugars, and a smart parent will take full advantage of this asset. In this book, I'll help you understand the benefits of using alternative cooking methods with several different ingredients. In some instances I've duplicated recipes and only changed the method of cooking. Amazingly, by varying the cooking method you will create a whole new flavor for your child, significantly reducing the hissy-fit factor. I know you know what I mean.

After trying a few recipes in this book, I think you'll find the following:

- You'll be able to create great-tasting, nutritious meals for your children and yourself, with a minimum of effort.
- You'll have learned a few simple techniques that will help you create a variety of delicious flavors and pleasing textures using very few ingredients. For example, who would have thought the combination of pork tenderloin, fresh peaches and sweet onions would emulate the flavor of authentic Southern barbecue?
- By paying attention to my "Not Just for Babies" tips you'll discover how to use the recipes you create for your kids as the basis for mouthwatering dishes geared to adult tastes. For example, I'll show you how to transform a basic carrot purée into Hawaiian Coconut Carrot Ginger Soup (see recipe, page 44).

I have included a fairly wide range of recipes, from basic, single-ingredient dishes to those that are more advanced, including Jonah's personal favorite, Fennel and Apple-Stuffed Pork Chops (see recipe, page 158). Just writing that sentence, I marvel at how refined Jonah's palate has become. When we're shopping for food, I'm always amazed at his requests — "that rack of lamb" from the butcher counter or "those ogre-anic grapes" in the organic section of the store. But that's the goal, isn't it? If you introduce your kids to a variety of nutritionally balanced good-tasting meals when they are very young, they'll develop healthy eating habits that will serve them well for the rest of their lives.

Now, if you'll excuse me, I've gotta go. Jonah and I are expecting company for dinner. Bon appetit!

— *Jordan Wagman*

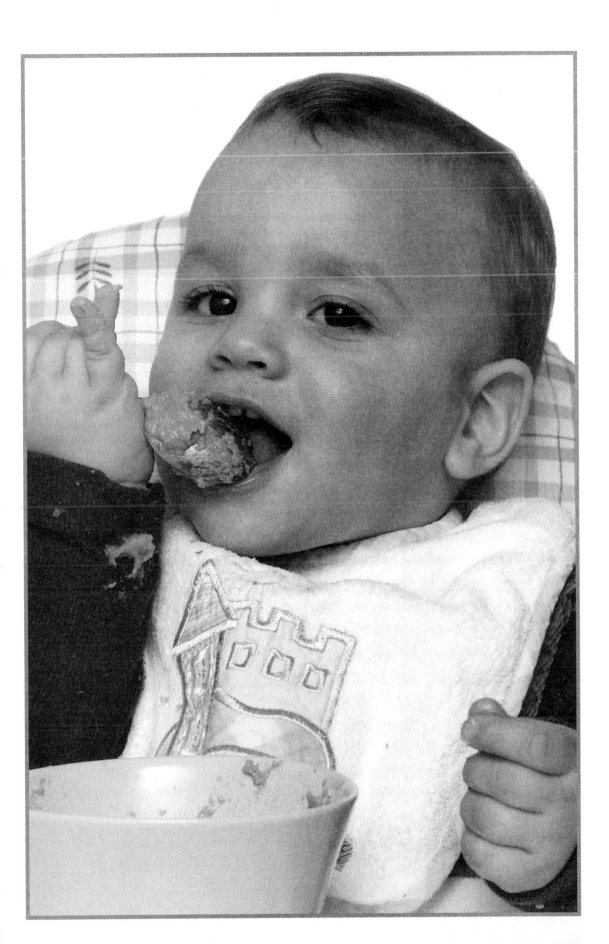

From the Nutritionist

As a nutritionist, I have a passion for food — both talking about it and eating it. I believe that a nutritious diet is our most valuable tool for promoting our families' health on a daily basis. Every time we feed our children we have an opportunity not only to nourish their bodies but also to expand their world.

I was thrilled when Jordan asked me to participate in this book. As a mother first and a nutritionist second, I completely understand the time pressures on family life and the draw of ready-made foods. However, I strongly believe that as a society our biggest problem from a nutritional perspective is our increasing reliance on refined and processed foods. For decades, these foods have been displacing fresh vegetables, fruits, whole grains, good fats and proteins in our diets. As rising rates of obesity and degenerative diseases such as type-2 diabetes suggest, we have done so at the expense of our health.

Our eating habits develop early in life. Preparing your own baby food from fresh, whole ingredients will help get your baby off to the best start possible because you are shaping her tastes and preferences in a positive direction. By using a wide variety of foods you are doing more than expanding her palate and creating new experiences with food; you are also ensuring that her diet is nutritious.

Why Make Your Own?

For optimal growth and development, a baby's body needs a sufficient supply of fresh water, carbohydrates, fats and proteins as well as dozens of essential vitamins and minerals. In recent years we've learned more and more about certain compounds called phytochemicals in fruits, vegetables and whole grains that also have health-promoting properties. The best way to provide these nutrients for your child is to serve him a balanced and varied diet based on whole foods that are minimally processed. And the best way to do that is by making your own baby food, using the freshest, best-quality ingredients you can find.

When ingredients such as vegetables are processed, they lose many of their essential nutrients. For instance, many commercially prepared baby foods contain additives that can affect the nutrient content of the food. A report by the Center for Science in the Public Interest compared fresh apricots with jarred ones from a leading baby food manufacturer. They knew that according to the USDA Food Database, one 4-ounce serving of fresh apricots provides about 335 mg of potassium and 2860 IU of vitamin A. By contrast, they found that one 4-ounce serving of the jarred baby food contained only 139 mg of potassium and 1333 IU of vitamin A, a considerable difference. (To prepare your baby a wholesome fresh apricot purée, see our recipe on page 37.) Thickening agents such as modified tapioca starch and wheat and potato starches, as well as added sugars and water, greatly dilute the nutrient content of prepared baby foods, making them nutritionally inferior to those made entirely from whole foods. Some commercial baby foods even contain salt and high-fructose corn syrup, which can have negative effects later in life, such as an increased risk for heart disease and obesity. Worse still, prepared baby foods are also more expensive than those you make at home.

Because children's dietary preferences are set early in life, it's important to predispose them to having a taste for whole healthy food rather than a preference for salty or heavily sweetened processed food. When you make your own baby food, you know exactly what your baby is eating. The added value is you can shape her taste for the better by limiting ingredients that may have potentially negative effects over the long term. Moreover, an early diet based on nutritious whole foods will help develop a healthy eater, one with a broad palate who will enjoy a wide variety of foods, while ensuring she obtains the full range of nutrients she needs for optimal development. The recipes in *Easy Gourmet Baby Food* stress the importance of whole foods and fresh ingredients. They also use a variety of foods, because variety is the foundation of a balanced healthy diet.

Enjoy Meals as a Family

Babies are social creatures who enjoy and thrive on the company of others throughout the day, including mealtime. Like most of us, they enjoy eating with other people more than eating alone. That's one reason why we have included information on how to transform the recipes for babies into dishes that Mom and Dad can enjoy as well. Not only are we trying to provide the best nutrition possible, we're also encouraging the entire family to eat together. A family meal is an opportunity for you as a parent to model healthy eating habits that your baby will notice and emulate later on. The very act of sitting down and eating with your children may also encourage them to eat what is offered and, if they see you enjoying them, to try foods they haven't had before. Studies show that regularly having dinner together as a family has numerous benefits, such as improved nutritional intake, a decreased risk for unhealthy weight and better emotional health. They also show that children who usually join their families at mealtime do better in school and are less likely to engage in high-risk behavior such as using drugs. Remember, a family meal doesn't have to be in the evening. Why not enjoy a breakfast smoothie and fruit purée with your baby?

What about organics?

Organic foods are defined as those produced without conventional pesticides, herbicides, antibiotics, growth hormones, irradiation or genetic engineering. In recent years, sales of organic foods have increased dramatically. Although people consider eating organic foods for many reasons, more than 90 per cent of people who actually purchase organics do so with a view toward reducing their exposure to pesticides. This is especially true for parents making decisions about the first foods to feed a baby. This makes sense. Babies and children may be more vulnerable to pesticide residues in food and drink because, among other factors, pound for pound, they eat more than adults. And because their diet is less varied than that of a typical adult, if one of the foods in their relatively small repertoire is particularly high in pesticide residue, their intake will be greater in relative terms.

Another reason why babies may be more susceptible to potential carcinogens from pesticides is that from conception through the first three or so years of his life, a baby's cells are multiplying at their peak and his vital organs and nervous system are developing. However, the key organs that assist the body in chemical detoxification — the liver and kidneys — are still immature and less able to break down and metabolize harmful substances.

So perhaps not surprisingly, in a risk assessment forum that took place in March 2005, the United States Environmental Protection Agency concluded that, on average, carcinogens are 10 times more potent for babies than for adults.

Pesticides in Produce

Over the past 15 years, the U.S. Department of Agriculture's (USDA) Pesticide Data Program has analyzed pesticides in about 200,000 food samples and has found residue from one or more pesticides in almost 80 per cent of the conventional produce tested. More than 90 per cent of conventionally grown strawberries, peaches, pears and apples have been shown to have pesticide residues. Perhaps surprisingly, some organically grown produce also contains residues, for a number of reasons. For instance, when a field is sprayed with pesticides from an aircraft, not all of the pesticide makes it to the ground. The wind can carry the spray to organic farms that may be miles away. Despite the rigorous certification programs organic farms go through to remain chemical-free, the soil may contain residues of insecticides such as DDT that still persist in the environment even though they have been banned for many years. These are called Persistent Organic Pollutants, or POPs, and they were banned when they were found to have a devastating effect on the health of wildlife and humans.

The good news is that although organic produce is not immune to pesticide residue, it appears in much smaller quantities. USDA testing done in 2004 showed that 16 per cent of the organic samples tested contained pesticide residues — less than one-quarter the incidence in conventionally grown produce. Other studies conducted by the USDA's Pesticide Data Program

"The Dirty Dozen"

The 12 fruits and vegetables containing the most pesticide residue, from most to least, are:

- peaches
- apples
- bell peppers
- celery
- nectarines
- strawberries
- cherries
- lettuce
- grapes (imported from outside the U.S.)
- pears
- spinach
- potatoes

Look for our "Buy Organic" message in the Nutrition Tip, which reminds you that the fruit or vegetable mentioned in the recipe is one of the 12 containing the most pesticide residue unless it is organically grown.

---

indicate that when chemical pesticides are present on organic produce, the average levels are substantially lower than the same pesticide on conventionally grown produce.

In 2006 a research group at the University of Washington in Seattle conducted the first dietary intervention study to examine the level of toxins in conventionally grown and organic foods. Twenty-three school-aged children were tested for organophosphate (OP) insecticides before eating a diet of organic food, while they were on the organic diet, and again after returning to a diet of conventionally produced food. All the children tested positive for OP toxins in their urine when they were eating conventionally produced food, but within five days of eating the all-organic diet, the OP levels virtually disappeared.

However, there is, to date, very little data, let alone consensus, on the potential risks from eating fruits and vegetables containing pesticide residues. Using thousands of pesticide analyses done between 2002 and 2004 by the USDA and the U.S. Food and Drug Administration, the Environmental Working Group (EWG), a U.S. nonprofit organization, has ranked the 43 most commonly eaten fruits and vegetables to determine those containing the most pesticide residues. They state that you can lower your pesticide exposure by almost 90 per cent if you avoid the 12 most contaminated fruits and vegetables and eat the 12 least contaminated ones instead. You can also buy organic versions of those belonging to the "dirty dozen" group.

Whichever way you determine is right for you, be assured that according to the U.S. National Cancer Institute, the risk of heart disease and many cancers is greatly reduced in people who eat more fruit and vegetables — with or without pesticides — than those who eat less. So please don't avoid the produce section of your local grocery store because it doesn't sell organic fruits and vegetables.

Avoid Pesticide Residues

Use this list to prioritize your options when you're thinking about purchasing organic produce for you and your baby. You will probably want to buy organic versions of the "dirty dozen," but may find nonorganic versions of the "consistently clean" acceptable.

Nutrient Content of Produce

Some studies have focused on the nutrient content of organic versus conventionally grown produce. One of the longest is the Long-Term Research on Agricultural Systems Project (LTRAS) conducted at the University of California, Davis. In June 2007, the study team reported that over a 10 year period, the level of quercetin, a phytonutrient that appears to have many healthful benefits, had increased 79 per cent in tomatoes as a result of organic management of the land. During the study, the quercetin level of the organic tomatoes increased yearly. However, the largest increase came after the land had been organically managed for seven years, suggesting that potential long-term nutritional benefits are linked with sustainable organic farming.

Meat and Poultry

When purchasing meat, poultry, eggs and dairy products there are a number of things to think about, such as whether the animals have been fed antibiotics routinely, rather than just to treat disease, or if their feed contained pesticides. Most pesticides are fat-soluble, meaning they accumulate in the fat of the animals that eat food with pesticide residue and also at the top of the food chain, in the fat of the humans eating those animals. Therefore, meat, dairy and eggs from conventionally raised livestock contain concentrated amounts of pesticides from the feed they have eaten over their lifespan. When we eat these products we ingest those residues.

Another concern is that large meat-producing farms that raise livestock conventionally are likely to use antibiotics subtherapeutically. This means they feed their animals antibiotics to prevent disease as well as to treat it, which is problematic. Through a chain of events, this practice can lead to the creation of drug-resistant bacteria, a serious emerging problem. Regulations put in place by the FDA, USDA and the Canadian Food Inspection Agency now require conventional farmers to stop giving their animals

"The Consistently Clean"

The 12 least contaminated fruits and vegetables from lowest to highest pesticide load are:

- onions
- avocado
- sweet corn
- pineapples
- mango
- sweet peas
- asparagus
- kiwi
- bananas
- cabbage
- broccoli
- eggplant

antibiotics for a regulated period of time before their meat, milk or eggs, in the case of poultry, are brought to market. This "withdrawal time" is specific to the antibiotic given and is designed to reduce any antibiotic residues that may be present.

In the United States there is also concern around genetically engineered recombinant bovine growth hormone (rBGH) that is injected into dairy cows to increase their milk production. Milk from these cows contains substantially more of a compound called insulin-like growth factor-1 (IGF-1), a naturally occurring hormone in both cows and humans. Elevated IGF-1 levels are a known risk factor for breast, colon and prostate cancers. Approximately 20 per cent of all dairy cows in the U.S. are injected with this hormone, although its use is banned in Canada and Europe.

Organically raised animals (and poultry) cannot be treated with growth hormones or antibiotics and must be given feed that has been produced organically. If an animal becomes ill and requires antibiotics, it is isolated from the rest of the herd and treated, but its meat and milk (or eggs in the case of poultry) cannot be certified as organic.

Raw Foods And Your Baby

Including raw fruits and vegetables in your baby's diet is an important feature of a well-rounded diet and has a number of health benefits. Raw, or "live," foods, as some people call them, contain plant enzymes that function as phytochemical nutrients in our bodies and help maximize your growing baby's health. They are also necessary for healthy bowel function and can contain higher levels of vitamins than their cooked counterparts.

On the other hand, cooking some vegetables can actually increase the body's ability to use certain nutrients. This includes some carotenoids — the lycopene in tomatoes and beta-carotene in carrots. However, many vitamins are water-soluble, in which case, they lose some of their impact in cooking. In order to minimize this loss, we recommend that you save the water from cooked vegetables and use it to thin your baby's first purées and other dishes. This way you are retaining some of the vitamins that were displaced.

Raw fruits and vegetables may harbor harmful bacteria like *E. coli*. So when you are preparing a recipe using raw food, make sure to be particularly careful when washing your produce.

Soy

Depending upon your source, soy is either a wonder food or one that is harmful to your health. Soy has been the subject of a plethora of studies, many of which provide conflicting results. The truth probably lies somewhere in between. Our perspective on soy revolves around the value of eating whole foods and the health benefits associated with eating a wide variety of foods. We believe that soy can be a very healthful part of a well-balanced and varied diet. We like to use it as organic tofu or as a whole food (edamame), bearing in mind, as with most foods, that too much of a good thing is still too much.

Essential Omega-3 Fatty Acids

"Low fat" has been an anti-obesity mantra for almost 30 years. Whether it is valid for adults is a subject of some debate, but a low-fat diet is definitely not appropriate for babies. During infancy and childhood an adequate supply of fat is essential. Fat is "energy-dense," supplying nine calories per gram compared with the four calories provided by the same amount of protein and carbohydrate. It is also necessary to consume fat so your body can absorb the fat-soluble vitamins A, D, E and K. And, perhaps not surprisingly, since our brains are more than 60 per cent fat, a sufficient amount of this nutrient is necessary for healthy brain development. Be conscious about not restricting natural fats for the first three or so years of your baby's life. However, trans fats that result from the process of hydrogenation, and which are prevalent in processed foods, are not healthy fats and do not belong in anyone's diet.

One of the most important fats for your baby is omega-3 essential fatty acids. These fats are called essential because the body can't make them. Consequently, they must be obtained from the diet.

Omega-3 fats are unsaturated and highly unstable. That means they degrade quickly with exposure to heat, light and oxygen and, as a result, are usually removed from processed foods, such as refined grains, with a view toward increasing the shelf life of products. For instance, Canadian consumers were recently surprised to learn that much of the flour sold in their country as "whole wheat" actually has up to 70 per cent of the bran and the germ (where the healthful oils reside) removed to help reduce rancidity and prolong shelf life.

Because omega-3 fatty acids must come from food, it is important to know where to find them. By far the best source is cold-water fish, such as salmon, halibut, herring, mackerel and sardines. Sometimes fish is not recommended for babies under 12 months because it is a potential allergen, but if there aren't any fish allergies in your family, it is a very good source of protein and can be added in the six- to nine-month range. Once your baby is a year old, you can certainly add fish to her diet.

The best vegetable sources of omega-3 fatty acids are flax seed oil, canola oil, walnut oil and hemp oil. Most nuts and seeds are a good source of omega-3s but they are not usually recommended for children younger than two, because they, too, are potential allergens. So how do you get these crucial nutrients into your baby? If you have concerns because your family has a history of allergies, consult your pediatrician. Otherwise, try adding a small amount ($\frac{1}{16}$ to $\frac{1}{8}$ teaspoon) of organic flax oil to your baby's favorite purée once a day for the first few days, after which time you can increase it to $\frac{1}{4}$ of a teaspoon once or twice a day. If you breastfeed your baby, the fat in your breast milk will reflect the fat in your diet, so do your baby and yourself a favor and increase your consumption of omega-3 fats. Not only are omega-3 fatty acids crucial for your baby, they are also beneficial for all age groups and appear to be helpful in improving a wide range of conditions, from arthritis to Alzheimer's disease. If you feed your baby formula, consider using one with high DHA (one of the omega-3 fats) content.

The omega-6 fatty acid, linoleic acid, is also an essential fatty acid that must be obtained from the diet. While it is important, it is not in short supply in a typical North American diet. Linoleic acid is readily available in foods such as whole grains, poultry, eggs, nuts and vegetable oils, such as corn and safflower oil.

One important thing to know about omega-3 and omega-6 fats is that they need to be taken into the body in the proper ratio. This ratio is about 2 to 1 of omega-6 to omega-3 fats. Unfortunately, most diets in North America are skewed to a 10 to 20 to 1 ratio of omega-6 to omega-3 fats, partially due to the processing of our foods. That's why it is important to consciously add omega-3-rich foods to your diet and that of your baby. Too much omega-6 fat may interfere with the absorption of omega-3 fats. An abundance of omega-6 fats is also part of a metabolic pathway in the body that can result in the production of inflammatory compounds that are detrimental to health.

Iron

Iron is a mineral your body needs. It helps form healthy red blood cells and is the central component of hemoglobin, which carries oxygen in the blood. During pregnancy, your baby built up the iron stores he needs to help fuel his considerable growth in the first year of life. At about the six-month mark, these stores start to decline and your baby's food must now become the source of necessary iron. Inadequate iron intake can increase the risk of iron-deficiency anemia and affect a child's development and learning ability early in life.

There are two different types of iron that can be used by the body. One, called heme iron, is found in meat and eggs. Foods rich in heme iron include meat and poultry (including duck). The other type, non-heme iron, is found in plants. Plant sources rich in iron include tofu, quinoa, barley, figs, apricots and all legumes. The iron from animal products is more easily absorbed by the body than iron from plant sources, but you can greatly increase the absorption of non-heme iron by ensuring that you consume foods that are high in vitamin C along with plant foods containing iron. Good amounts of vitamin C can be found in apples, broccoli, Brussels sprouts, sweet potatoes, red peppers and tomatoes.

Omega-3 Fats and ADHD

In recent years researchers have been looking at how omega-3 fats affect brain function, specifically in association with attention deficit hyperactivity disorder (ADHD). The results of a recent study published in the *Journal of Developmental and Behavioral Pediatrics* supported the link between ADHD and deficiencies in omega-3 fats. In this study, school-aged children were given capsules containing either palm oil or omega-3 fats, and their behavior was followed for 15 weeks. The children who received the omega-3 capsules showed improvement in the core symptoms of inattention, hyperactivity and impulsivity, compared with those who received palm oil.

Use Whole, Not Refined Grains

The iron in whole grains is found in the bran and the germ of the grain. When these grains are refined and milled, as they are in commercially prepared baby cereals, approximately 75 per cent of the naturally occurring iron is lost. As a result, the iron that was removed needs to be added back through the process of fortification. In *Easy Gourmet Baby Food* we have provided you with many whole-grain options that can be used instead of commercially-prepared cereals. Try Simple Barley Cereal (see recipe, page 52), Basic Quinoa (see recipe, page 48), Brown Rice Cereal (see recipe, page 50), Simple Millet Cereal (see recipe, page 49), Whole-Grain Oat Cereal with Grapes (see recipe, page 53), Quinoa and Banana Purée (see recipe, page 54) or Apple and Fig Brown Rice Cereal (see recipe, page 56).

The Vegetarian Baby

Vegetarianism, which has been part of various cultures for millennia, is becoming increasingly popular in North America as a lifestyle choice. There are two basic ways of being a vegetarian. Vegans don't eat animal products at all, including eggs and dairy, while lacto-ovo vegetarians eat dairy products and eggs but no meat, poultry, fish or seafood. Becoming a vegetarian may be a moral or ethical decision, but many adults have based their choice on the well-researched benefits of a plant-based diet and the reduction of animal fats.

Even so, being a vegetarian doesn't necessarily mean a person has a nutritious and healthful diet. It takes careful planning to ensure that the foods you eat are nutritionally adequate. In choosing a vegetarian diet for your baby, you'll need to understand the fundamentals of carbohydrates, proteins, fats and vitamins and minerals to ensure your baby receives optimal nutrition. It is important to know the best source of critical nutrients such as iron, calcium, vitamin B_{12} and vitamin D, all of which are easier to find in animal foods.

Allergies

The immaturity of a baby's digestive system makes him more susceptible to both food intolerances and allergies. That's why it is best to introduce your baby to a single purée for five to seven days before adding another new food. This is especially important if there is a family history of food allergies. Using just one food for a few days will help you recognize which foods, if any, your baby may not be able to tolerate or that cause an allergic reaction. A food allergy occurs when the baby's immune system tries to defend his body against a food it has identified as "foreign," by producing antibodies. Repeated exposure to an allergen is generally required for the body to produce enough antibodies to cause an allergic reaction. Symptoms such as skin rashes, hives, a runny nose, itching, congestion, wheezing, abdominal pain and poor weight gain can characterize an allergic reaction. The most serious allergic reaction is anaphylaxis (mouth or throat swelling, difficulty breathing) which is life-threatening and requires immediate emergency medical attention. Anaphylaxis generally happens either immediately after exposure to the allergen or within a number of hours. Less serious reactions may also be immediate but they can also be delayed for up to two days. Once you have determined that your child doesn't react to a certain food, you can combine it with other foods that you know won't cause a reaction.

In this introduction I have touched on some of the nutrition issues that are important for your baby. I have also included a nutrition tip with each recipe to help you understand the inherent value of whole foods and to provide you with more detailed information about how to use them in your day-to-day life. While each tip usually focuses on a particular aspect of one of the ingredients in the recipe, I hope you will use the information to expand your knowledge of nutrition. Share it with your baby (they are never too young to start learning!). Mostly I hope it helps you to appreciate that whole foods are meant to nourish us and be enjoyed.

Feeding a baby is a wonderful experience, although at times it can be frustrating. Try to relax and enjoy the process. Remember, when you make your own baby food from natural wholesome ingredients, you are starting your child out on a pattern of healthy eating that will have lifelong benefits.

— *Jill Hillhouse*
B.P.H.E., R.N.C.P.
Registered Holistic Nutritionist

Preparing Your Own Baby Food

This book is about preparing food for your baby that tastes very, very good — so good, in fact, that you'll want to share it. The starting point for producing the best-tasting meals is the freshest (ideally locally produced) ingredients. Often they are very simply prepared. While there is no shame in making or buying meals for your kids because it's convenient, with the right ingredients, a little bit of planning and recipes in this book, you can feed your family the kinds of meals you always wanted to but didn't think you had the time to make. And you can do it without spending your days trapped in the kitchen. We know you want to give your baby a great start by preparing your own delicious and nutritious foods, so keep these things in mind before you start.

Keep It Clean

Because your baby's gastrointestinal tract (a key component of her immune system) isn't mature, she is more susceptible to food-borne illnesses, which are caused by ingesting foods contaminated with bacteria, viruses and chemical toxins. It's your job as a parent to minimize these risks, so before starting to prepare your baby's food, wash your hands thoroughly for at least 20 seconds with warm water and soap. Thorough hand washing is the single most important thing you can do to prevent illness. Once your hands are clean, make sure that all your equipment, cooking utensils and all work surfaces have also been thoroughly washed with hot water and soap.

Avoid Cross-Contamination

Cross-contamination refers to the transfer of harmful bacteria among foods. To avoid this possibility, keep raw meat, fish and poultry separate from produce. Use separate cutting boards for these foods and pay particular attention to washing any utensils and cutting boards that have come into contact with them in hot soapy water immediately after use. After washing, sanitize using a solution of 1 tsp (5 mL) of chlorine bleach combined with 3 cups (750 mL) hot water. Be sure you rinse everything thoroughly to remove the bleach and then leave the equipment to air dry.

Wash Fruits, Vegetables and Grains

As many as 20 people may have touched the produce you're feeding to your baby, so be sure to wash it well. The best way to remove surface dirt and bacteria (and, if you're using conventionally grown produce, some of the pesticide residue) is to rub it briskly with your hands under cool or warm running water. Even if you plan to peel it, thoroughly scrub produce that has rinds, grooves or waxy skins (such as melons, cucumber, squash, citrus, potatoes and even bananas) with a vegetable brush. Because cutting through the rind can transfer dirt and bacteria to the fleshy part inside, you want the surface to be as clean as possible. Place loose berries and bunched fruit such as grapes and blueberries in a colander and rinse under running water or with a spray nozzle. Even organic and prewashed vegetables need to be washed before consumption to eliminate any potential contamination caused by human handling.

Whole grains should also be washed before use. Most have been at least partially cleaned before they get to market but require a further cleansing to eliminate any dust and fine particles that may stick to the kernels. Some grains, such as quinoa, have a natural coating called saponin, which, although harmless, may impart a bitter taste to the cooked product. To wash whole grains, place them in a large bowl and add approximately three times their volume of water. Gently rub the kernels with your hands, loosening any debris. Transfer to a fine mesh strainer and rinse under cool running water until the water runs clear.

Storing and Freezing Cooked Food

Improperly stored food can be another source of food-borne illness. If your baby does not eat all of the food you have prepared for her, transfer it to a clean container, cover and store in the refrigerator for up to three days. If you don't plan to use all of it within that time frame, freeze at least a portion immediately.

Avoid Commercial Produce Washes

We do not recommend washing produce with detergent, antibacterial soap or bleach solutions. These products may contain chemicals that are not intended for use on foods, which porous fruits and vegetables can absorb. The Federal Department of Agriculture (FDA) in the United States does not recommend using commercial produce sprays or washes because their effectiveness has not been standardized.

Don't wait until the food has been in the fridge for three days to freeze it.

To freeze, pour cooled food into a clean ice cube tray, cover with foil and place in the freezer. Once the food is frozen solid (within 24 hours) turn out the serving-size frozen cubes into a freezer bag and label with the date and the contents. You can keep food safely frozen for up to three months. Freezing will preserve most of the nutrients in your homemade baby food.

Thawing

Always thaw frozen baby food in a sealed container in the fridge or in the top of a double boiler on the stove. Thawing on the countertop at room temperature can promote bacterial growth that could be unsafe for your baby. Throw away any food that has not been eaten after it has been thawed. Do not refreeze any baby food. We don't recommend using a microwave for thawing or heating baby food or bottles. There is a danger of hot spots in the food that could burn your baby's mouth or throat.

Recommended Equipment

The following is a list of the basic kitchen equipment you will need to create these delicious recipes for your baby.

- immersion blender or all-purpose blender
- potato masher
- whisk
- heat-proof rubber spatula
- wooden spoon
- tongs
- colander
- sharp knives
- skillet
- ovenproof sauté pan and saucepan
- pepper grinder
- ice cube trays
- freezer bags

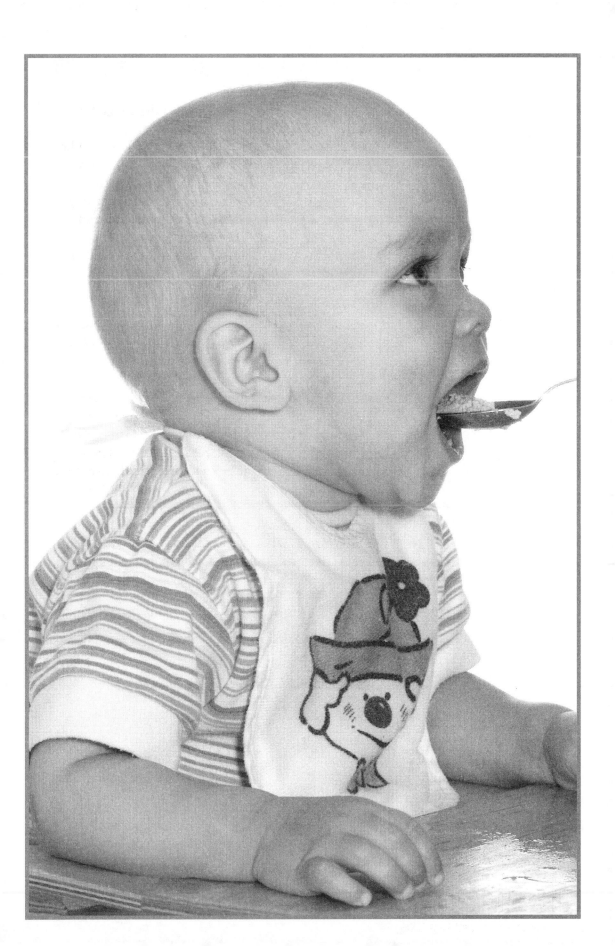

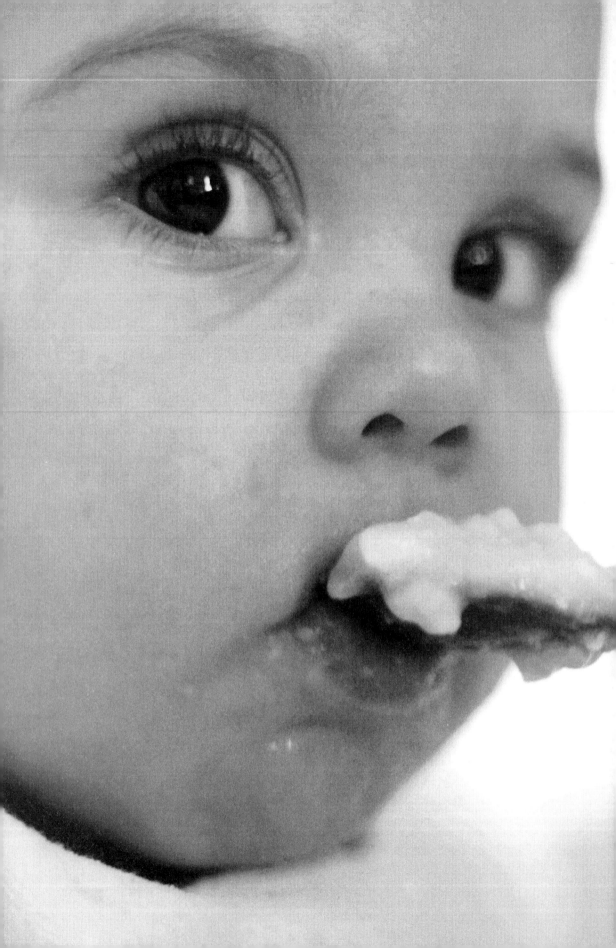

Starting Solids
(6 to 9 Months)

Introduction 32

Single Fruits
Roasted Banana Purée 34
Apple Medley. 35
Bosc Pear Purée 36
Fresh Apricot Purée. 37
Blueberry Purée 38
Mango Purée 39

Single Vegetables
Broccoli Purée 40
Sweet Potato Purée 41
Roasted Sweet Potato Purée. 42
Acorn Squash Purée 43
Carrot Purée. 44
Sweet Pea Purée. 45
Roasted Beet Purée 46
Caramelized Parsnip Purée 47

Single Grains
Basic Quinoa 48
Simple Millet Cereal 49
Brown Rice Cereal 50
Simple Barley Cereal. 52

Grains and Fruit
Whole-Grain Oat Cereal
   with Grapes 53
Quinoa and Banana Purée 54
Apple and Fig Brown Rice Cereal 56

Other Combos
Tofu, Bosc Pears and Banana 57
Roasted Apple, Blueberry
   and Pear. 58
Nectarine and Carrot Purée 59
Apricot Acorn Squash Purée 60
Green Bean Purée with
   Fresh Basil 61
Honeydew, Blueberry and
   Mint Purée 62
Plum and Blueberry Purée. 63
Zucchini and Basil Purée. 64
Cauliflower and Parsnip Purée 65
Cauliflower and Chickpea
   Chowder. 66
Banana and Blueberry Purée. 67
Carrot and Split Pea Purée 68
Watermelon, Peach and
   Blueberry Purée. 69
Avocado, Carrot and Cucumber
   Purée 70
Red Lentil and Apple 71

Meat and Legumes
Celery Root and Chicken Purée. 72
Sweet Peas, Lamb and Parsnip 73
Chicken and Red Lentils 74
Grilled Chicken and Avocado 75
White Navy Bean and Beef
   Tenderloin Purée. 76

Introduction

Don't Stop Breast or Bottle Feeding

Remember, while you are introducing first foods, continue breast or formula feeding because these are still the best sources of nutrition for your growing baby.

For about the first six months of life, your baby will get the nutrients he or she needs from either breast milk or iron-fortified infant formula. At the six-month point, the American Academy of Pediatrics and the Canadian Pediatric Society recommend starting solid foods as a complement to breast milk or formula. This is a very exciting time for both you and your baby. You are helping to expand your baby's horizons as together you begin to explore the fascinating world of food.

Every baby develops and progresses at his individual pace. You know your baby best, so be patient and take your time. Watch for the following signs that indicate your baby may be ready for "people food."

- Your baby is interested in the foods you are eating and may try to reach for them.
- Your baby can sit by himself or with minimal support and hold his head up well.
- Your baby opens his mouth when he sees food coming toward his face. He can close his mouth over a small spoon rather than pushing it out with his tongue.
- Your baby wants to feed more often, or seems to want more after breast or bottle feeds.
- Your baby is beginning to make a chewing motion with his mouth.
- Your baby can turn away or push food away with his hands.

At six months your baby's gastrointestinal tract will be mature enough to handle solid foods. He will also begin to need the additional nutrients provided by whole foods. Your pediatrician will likely recommend beginning with a single-grain, iron-fortified infant cereal. Subsequently, introduce single foods, one at a time, waiting five to seven days before trying a new one.

This way, you will be able to identify any foods that cause adverse reactions. Plain foods that do not contain added salt, sugar or spices are preferable at this stage of development.

It is important that your baby's first foods contain iron to fuel his rapid growth. Foods that contain iron include cooked egg yolks, poultry, meat, tofu and legumes. Some fruits and vegetables also contain a type of iron whose absorption is increased by the presence of vitamin C (see page 23).

Contrary to what you may have heard, starting your baby with fruit will not nurture a sweet tooth, because breast milk itself is quite sweet. In this chapter we offer single cereals, fruits and vegetables to get your baby started. After working your way through these single foods and learning which your baby can tolerate and prefers, you can move on to try various combinations you think he will enjoy.

Introducing your baby to solid food is more of an art than a science, and a messy one at that. Allow your baby to enjoy his food and don't be too worried about exactly how much he is actually eating. At first most will end up in his hair or on the floor anyway.

In this chapter we have developed a wide variety of single and double food purées to help you introduce your baby to a diverse assortment of nutrients and tastes. Every baby is unique and develops his own preferences for food. Just because your baby turns away the first (or tenth) time you offer a particular food doesn't mean you should stop trying. Your baby's palate will change and develop if given the opportunity. A food he once wouldn't touch may well become next month's favorite.

The preferred consistency of food will also vary from baby to baby and from month to month. If your baby prefers his food to be a slightly runny, thin it with breast milk or formula, or use the cooking water from recipes. This will help to maximize nutrient intake.

Roasted Banana Purée

The smell of roasted bananas will permeate beyond the kitchen, and your neighbors will be knocking down your door asking to taste what you've got cooking. Oh, your baby will love this yummy concoction, too!

Makes about 1 cup (250 mL)

▪ ▪ ▪

Chef Jordan's Tips

For the sweetest purée, use overripe bananas. This is a great way to use up any bananas you may have sitting around.

Always take care when adding hot liquids to a blender. Fill the container no more than half full or allow to cool before blending.

Nutrition Tip

As a first food bananas are smooth and easy to swallow. Because they are sweet, like breast milk and formula, your baby will take to them easily. If your baby has diarrhea or vomiting, the potassium in bananas helps to replenish the mineral balance in her body. Bananas also have an astringent or drying property, which may help reduce the water loss associated with diarrhea.

• Preheat oven to 250°F (120°C)

2	bananas, unpeeled (about 12 oz/375 g) (see Tips, left)	2
½ cup	water	125 mL

1. Place bananas on baking sheet and roast in preheated oven until soft, about 30 minutes. Transfer bananas to a plate and transfer cooking liquid from the baking sheet to a saucepan. Set aside and let bananas cool until they can be easily handled.

2. Peel cooled bananas, holding them over the saucepan to catch the liquid, then add to the saucepan. Add water and bring to a boil over medium heat. Remove from heat and transfer to a blender or use an immersion blender in the saucepan. Purée until smooth. Let cool until warm to the touch or transfer to an airtight container and refrigerate for up to 3 days or freeze for up to 1 month.

Nutrients per serving (¼ cup/50 mL)	
Calories 53	Dietary fiber . . . . . . 1.5 g
Protein . . . . 0.6 g	Sodium . . . . 1.5 mg
Total fat . . . . 0.2 g	Calcium . . . . 3.9 mg
Saturated fat. . . . . . 0.1 g	Iron . . . . 0.2 mg
Carbohydrates. . . . 13.5 g	Vitamin C. . . . . . . 5.1 mg

Not just for babies
Mom and Dad will enjoy this purée warmed with a drop of cognac and drizzled over vanilla ice cream.

Apple Medley

In this recipe, the combination of sweet and sour apples builds a complex flavor profile. It's really worth the effort to use more than one type of apple.

Makes about 2 cups (500 mL)

■ ■ ■

Chef Jordan's Tips
The owner of one of the top French restaurants in southern California, Chef Pascal Olhats, would always remind me to "skim, skim, skim. Why would you want those impurities in your sauce?" he'd ask. In this recipe you should skim and discard the bubbles that rise to the top, which can make your purée bitter.

Nutrition Tip
Being concerned over the frequency and consistency of your infant's bowel movements is a natural state for parents of a new baby. Quite simply, all apples are great sources of both soluble and insoluble fiber, which are crucial for bowel health. The pectin in apples can help regulate both diarrhea and constipation.

Buy organic apples

1 cup	water	250 mL
1 cup	chopped cored Granny Smith or other tart apple (about 1)	250 mL
1 cup	chopped cored Gala or other sweet apple (about 1)	250 mL

1. In a saucepan, combine water, Granny Smith and Gala apples. Bring to a boil over medium heat. Reduce heat to low and simmer, skimming off any bubbles that rise to the top (see Tips, left), until apples are fork tender and water has reduced by three-quarters, 12 to 15 minutes.

2. Transfer to a blender or use an immersion blender in the saucepan. Purée until smooth. Let cool until warm to the touch or transfer to an airtight container and refrigerate for up to 3 days or freeze for up to 1 month.

Nutrients per serving (¼ cup/50 mL)

Calories	16	Dietary fiber	0.7 g
Protein	0.1 g	Sodium	1.2 mg
Total fat	0.0 g	Calcium	2.7 mg
Saturated fat	0.0 g	Iron	0.1 mg
Carbohydrates	4.3 g	Vitamin C	1.6 mg

Not just for babies
The addition of a pinch of cinnamon and brown sugar makes an excellent applesauce.

Bosc Pear Purée

This recipe brings back memories of my Gramma Jean's warm pear-apple sauce. Her recipe came all the way from Paducah, Ky., but it sure was a welcome treat on a cold winter's day in Toronto.

Makes about 2 cups (500 mL)

■ ■ ■

Chef Jordan's Tip
Often I'll choose to mix the same ingredient, cooked and raw (finely diced), before serving. I love the contrast in flavors (the cooked becomes so much sweeter) and textures. As your child is able to handle more texture, at about 8 or 9 months, try adding about ¼ cup (50 mL) peeled and diced raw pear for every 1 cup (250 mL) of purée.

Nutrition Tip
Pears are second only to bananas as a wonderful first food. They are an excellent source of fiber to help tone your baby's intestines and promote bowel health. Along with bananas, they have low allergenic potential, meaning they are not likely to cause any adverse reactions.

Buy organic pears

2¼ cups	chopped cored Bosc pears (about 3)	550 mL
1 cup	water	250 mL

1. In a saucepan, combine pears and water. Bring to a boil over medium heat. Reduce heat to low, cover, leaving a small crack to allow steam to escape, and simmer until pears are fork tender and most of the water has evaporated, about 15 minutes.

2. Transfer to a blender or use an immersion blender in the saucepan. Purée until smooth. Let cool until warm to the touch or transfer to an airtight container and refrigerate for up to 3 days or freeze for up to 1 month.

Nutrients per serving (¼ cup/50 mL)	
Calories 27	Dietary fiber . . . . . . 1.4 g
Protein . . . . 0.2 g	Sodium . . . . 1.4 mg
Total fat . . . . 0.1 g	Calcium . . . . 5.1 mg
Saturated fat. . . . . . 0.0 g	Iron . . . . 0.1 mg
Carbohydrates. . . . . 7.2 g	Vitamin C. . . . . . . 2.0 mg

Not just for babies
After scooping off an appropriate amount for your baby, add cinnamon to taste and 1 tbsp (15 mL) brown sugar to create a special treat reminiscent of my Gramma Jean's warm pear sauce.

Fresh Apricot Purée

This is one of my favorite purées. Fresh apricots are a real treat for anyone's palate.

**Makes about
1 cup (250 mL)**

▪ ▪ ▪

Chef Jordan's Tips

The quickest way to pit an apricot is to split it in half by hand and pull out the pit.

If fresh apricots aren't available, use the dried version. They yield a more gelatinous texture but a good flavor. Use 1 cup (250 mL) dried apricots in this recipe.

Nutrition Tip

If you are using dried apricots avoid the ones preserved with sulfites, which will likely be bright orange. Sulfites are a chemical preservative and are potentially toxic to developing bodies. They have been linked to allergic reactions and asthma. Look for apricots preserved with potassium sorbate or sorbic acid, which will look more brown than orange.

| 1½ cups | pitted apricots (about 10 oz/300 g) | 375 mL |
| ½ cup | water | 125 mL |

1. In a saucepan, combine apricots and water. Bring to a boil over medium heat. Cover, reduce heat to low and simmer until apricots are soft, about 15 minutes. Let cool to room temperature.

2. Transfer to a blender or use an immersion blender in the saucepan. Purée until smooth. Serve immediately or transfer to an airtight container and refrigerate for up to 3 days or freeze for up to 1 month.

Nutrients per serving (¼ cup/50 mL)

Calories	34	Dietary fiber	1.4 g
Protein	1.0 g	Sodium	1.6 mg
Total fat	0.3 g	Calcium	10.1 mg
Saturated fat	0.0 g	Iron	0.3 mg
Carbohydrates	7.9 g	Vitamin C	7.1 mg

Not just for babies

How about an apricot martini? One tablespoon (15 mL) of this purée added to a martini makes a refreshing drink for Mom and Dad.

Blueberry Purée

I realized I wanted to be a chef while camping in a wilderness park. As a teenager, I used to lead children on canoe trips, and one day we made pancakes using the wild blueberries we had picked. There is no better feeling than picking food from the wild and creating something people love. Thank you, blueberries!

Makes about 1 cup (250 mL)

| 2 cups | fresh or frozen blueberries | 500 mL |
| 1½ cups | water | 375 mL |

1. In a saucepan, combine blueberries and water. Bring to a boil over medium heat. Boil until berries are splitting in half, about 10 minutes.
2. Transfer to a blender or use an immersion blender in the saucepan. Purée until smooth. Let cool until warm to the touch, or transfer to an airtight container and refrigerate for up to 3 days or freeze for up to 1 month.

Chef Jordan's Tips

This purée tends to look thin while warm, but don't worry, it will thicken as it cools.

Nutrition Tip

Blueberries are small but mighty. They have a high ORAC value (oxygen radical absorbance capacity), which is the measure of their antioxidant level. Even though she still has a long way to go, feeding your baby foods with high ORAC values helps decrease the risk of degenerative disease that comes with aging. Wild blueberries are a particularly good choice because they have an ORAC value that is almost 50 per cent higher than farmed blueberries.

Nutrients per serving (¼ cup/50 mL)	
Calories 42	Dietary fiber . . . . . . 1.8 g
Protein . . . . 0.6 g	Sodium . . . . 3.4 mg
Total fat . . . . 0.2 g	Calcium . . . . 7.1 mg
Saturated fat. . . . . . 0.0 g	Iron . . . . 0.2 mg
Carbohydrates. . . . 10.7 g	Vitamin C. . . . . . . 7.2 mg

Not just for babies

Throughout the summer months my family often spends time at our cottage. Every weekend that Tamar and I are there we make a stuffed Brie cheese using this purée. Cut a 6-inch (15 cm) round of Brie in half horizontally and spread with about 2 tbsp (25 mL) of this purée. Wrap tightly in foil and bake in a 300°F (150°C) oven until soft, about 15 minutes.

Mango Purée

This is a particularly sweet-tasting purée with a fresh flavor that will appeal to everyone.

**Makes about
1¾ cups (425 mL)**

■ ■ ■

1	large mango (or 2 small), peeled, pitted and chopped (see Tips, left)	1
1 cup	water	250 mL

1. In a saucepan, combine mango and water. Bring to a boil over medium heat. Reduce heat to low and simmer until mango is soft, about 5 minutes.

2. Transfer to a blender or use an immersion blender in the saucepan. Purée until smooth. Let cool until warm to the touch or transfer to an airtight container and refrigerate for up to 3 days or freeze for up to 1 month.

Chef Jordan's Tips
The simplest way to peel a mango is with a regular vegetable peeler. Use a paring knife to cut away the flesh from the pit.

My father-in-law introduced me to the Atulfo mango. Golden yellow, it is the smallest of the mango varieties and is the most "buttery." If it's available, definitely choose this variety.

Nutrition Tip
Like all yellow, orange and red fruits, mangos are rich in beta-carotene, which your body makes into vitamin A. Vitamin A is required for skin cells to reproduce correctly. This helps them reduce the mutations that can lead to cancer. Good levels of vitamin A in your baby's body can help prevent diaper rash and outbreaks of eczema.

Nutrients per serving (¼ cup/50 mL)	
Calories 20	Dietary fiber . . . . . . 0.3 g
Protein . . . . 0.0 g	Sodium . . . . 1.1 mg
Total fat . . . . 0.1 g	Calcium . . . . 1.1 mg
Saturated fat. . . . . . 0.0 g	Iron . . . . 0.0 mg
Carbohydrates. . . . . 4.9 g	Vitamin C. . . . . . . 2.6 mg

Not just for babies
This purée is very versatile. Add it to your yogurt in the morning, use it as a basis for an afternoon power smoothie or drizzle over good-quality vanilla ice cream for dessert.

Broccoli Purée

If you and your family aren't fans of broccoli, wait until you try my purée. Just imagine broccoli purée that is a vibrant green color. That's because I keep my water at a rolling boil, which cooks it faster and maintains its color.

Makes about 1 cup (250 mL)

Chef Jordan's Tips

I use the term "fork tender" when teaching new cooks. It literally means to pierce a fork into something: if no resistance is felt, it's cooked. This is a wonderful point of reference.

Although fresh, locally grown broccoli is best, frozen broccoli florets are an adequate substitute in this recipe.

Nutrition Tip

Broccoli always makes the super food list. It is a nondairy source of calcium, an important mineral. During the rapid growth of infancy and toddlerhood your child needs calcium in significant amounts. Calcium not only optimizes the growth of her bones and teeth but also provides for healthy muscle contraction, including her heart.

| 4 cups | water | 1 L |
| 2 cups | broccoli florets | 500 mL |

1. In a saucepan, bring water to a rolling boil over high heat. Add broccoli. Cover and cook until broccoli is fork tender (see Tips, left), about 5 minutes. Strain through a colander set over a measuring cup or bowl, reserving the cooking liquid.

2. Transfer broccoli to a blender with 1 cup (250 mL) of reserved liquid or return to saucepan and use an immersion blender. Purée until smooth. Let cool until warm to the touch or transfer to an airtight container and refrigerate for up to 3 days or freeze for up to 1 month.

Nutrients per serving (¼ cup/50 mL)

Calories 10	Dietary fiber . . . . . . 1.0 g
Protein . . . . 1.1 g	Sodium . . . . 16.7 mg
Total fat . . . . 0.1 g	Calcium . . . . 24.1 mg
Saturated fat. . . . . . 0.0 g	Iron . . . . 0.3 mg
Carbohydrates. . . . . 1.9 g	Vitamin C. . . . . . 33.1 mg

Not just for babies

Add ⅓ cup (75 mL) of freshly grated Parmesan cheese to this purée to transform it into a great sauce to serve over long noodles like spaghetti or linguine.

Sweet Potato Purée

I'm sure that the natural sweetness of this tuber will be a huge hit with your baby — it's one of Jonah's favorites. Trust me, it will serve you well throughout the macaroni and cheese years (see Not just for babies, below).

**Makes about
2 cups (500 mL)**

■ ■ ■

Chef Jordan's Tips

I never puréed sweet potatoes with their skins until my wife, Tamar, and I began to create recipes for our company, Sweetpea Baby Food. Tamar asked me why I wasn't using the skins, and I had no good answer for her (I rarely do). I soon learned that sweet potatoes cooked with their skins have a much deeper flavor. But if you prefer, feel free to try the recipe without the skin.

Nutrition Tip

The skins of vegetables contain many of the nutrients. Skins are composed of cellulose, which contributes insoluble fiber, or roughage, to the diet. Fiber is important to the way your baby's food is digested and eliminated. Sweet potatoes, particularly their skins, also contain phenolic compounds, which are antioxidants.

| 2 | sweet potatoes, chopped (about 1 lb/500 g) (see Tips, left) | 2 |
| 1½ cups | water | 375 mL |

1. In a saucepan, combine sweet potatoes and water. Bring to a boil over medium heat. Reduce heat to low and simmer until potatoes are fork tender, about 15 minutes. Remove from heat.

2. Transfer potatoes and liquid to a blender or use an immersion blender in the saucepan. Purée until smooth. Let cool until warm to the touch or transfer to an airtight container and refrigerate for up to 3 days or freeze for up to 1 month.

Nutrients per serving (¼ cup/50 mL)	
Calories 35	Dietary fiber . . . . . . 1.2 g
Protein . . . . 0.6 g	Sodium . . . . 23.8 mg
Total fat . . . . 0.0 g	Calcium . . . . 13.6 mg
Saturated fat. . . . . . 0.0 g	Iron . . . . 0.3 mg
Carbohydrates. . . . . 8.2 g	Vitamin C. . . . . . . 1.0 mg

Not just for babies

My son, Jonah, hadn't eaten what most people call macaroni and cheese until he was about three. We served him sweet potato purée with Parmesan cheese over bow-tie noodles, and it has been his favorite lunch from his very first taste. Mom and Dad love it, too.

Roasted Sweet Potato Purée

This recipe produces a purée that is much more candy-like than the boiled version but with all the good nutrition.

**Makes about
2 cups (500 mL)**

■ ■ ■

Chef Jordan's Tips

Steeping the sweet potato in liquid while it cools softens the skins, smoothing the purée.

If butternut squash is in season substitute 1 small butternut squash for the sweet potato. Cook it whole and seed it after roasting. Purée with the skin left on for added flavor.

Nutrition Tip

Sweet potatoes are loaded with beta-carotene, a phytochemical found in all yellow, orange, red and dark green vegetables and fruits, and which your body breaks down to form vitamin A. Beta-carotene contains antioxidants, powerful scavengers that find and neutralize free radicals, which over time can contribute to disease. Eating richly colored fruits and vegetables on a daily basis helps minimize their long-term effects.

● Preheat oven to 350°F (180°C)

| 2 | sweet potatoes (about 1 lb/500 g) | 2 |
| 1 cup | water | 250 mL |

1. On a baking sheet, roast sweet potatoes in preheated oven until fork tender, about 1 hour.
2. Transfer sweet potatoes to a saucepan and add water. Bring to a boil over medium heat. Let cool to room temperature (see Tips, left).
3. Transfer to a blender or use an immersion blender in the saucepan. Purée until smooth. Serve immediately or transfer to an airtight container and refrigerate for up to 3 days or freeze for up to 1 month.

Nutrients per serving (¼ cup/50 mL)

Calories 35	Dietary fiber . . . . . . 1.2 g
Protein . . . . 0.6 g	Sodium . . . . 23.3 mg
Total fat . . . . 0.0 g	Calcium . . . . 13.1 mg
Saturated fat. . . . . . 0.0 g	Iron . . . . 0.3 mg
Carbohydrates. . . . . 8.2 g	Vitamin C. . . . . . . 1.0 mg

Not just for babies

The addition of 1 tsp (5 mL) unsalted butter and a pinch each of kosher salt and freshly ground black pepper makes an excellent side dish to accompany beef, pork or chicken.

Acorn Squash Purée

This simple purée, which is very versatile, provides the stuffing base for many ravioli dishes I've made. I often season it with sage and brown butter, a classic combination.

Makes about 1 cup (250 mL)

2½ cups	coarsely chopped peeled acorn squash (12 oz/375 g)	625 mL
2 cups	water	500 mL

Chef Jordan's Tips

The moisture content of squash can vary, so reserve the cooking liquid when straining. You may need it to thin out your purée. It's much tastier than water.

When shopping for acorn squash, choose one you can easily hold in your hand, about 5 to 6 inches (12.5 to 15 cm) around. These tend to be the sweetest.

Nutrition Tip

Darker-fleshed winter squash such as acorn, butternut and pumpkin have considerably higher amounts of beta-carotene (an antioxidant) than lighter-fleshed summer squash such as yellow zucchini, crookneck and straight-neck varieties. So as a general rule choose darkly pigmented fruits and vegetables for higher nutritional value.

1. In a saucepan, combine squash and water. Bring to a boil over medium heat. Reduce heat to low and simmer until squash is fork tender, about 25 minutes. In a colander set over a bowl, strain squash, reserving cooking liquid. Let cool to room temperature.

2. Transfer squash to a blender or return to saucepan and use an immersion blender. Purée squash until smooth, adding enough of the reserved liquid to reach desired consistency (see Tips, left). Let cool until warm to the touch or transfer to an airtight container and refrigerate for up to 3 days or freeze for up to 1 month.

Nutrients per serving (¼ cup/50 mL)

Calories	34	Dietary fiber	1.3 g
Protein	0.7 g	Sodium	6.1 mg
Total fat	0.1 g	Calcium	31.6 mg
Saturated fat	0.0 g	Iron	0.6 mg
Carbohydrates	8.9 g	Vitamin C	9.4 mg

Not just for babies

Enjoy the recipe as is. Serve alongside a whole roasted chicken or under a beef stew. Triple the recipe to have enough to feed Mom and Dad.

Carrot Purée

Carrots are a staple in our home, from baby yellow carrots to the larger everyday versions. Children love their natural sweetness.

Makes about 1 cup (250 mL)

■ ■ ■

Chef Jordan's Tips

I often roast carrots until caramelized, then purée them. The depth of flavor is unbelievable. Toss the chopped carrots in 1 tbsp (15 mL) extra virgin olive oil and roast in a preheated oven (300°F/150°C) until golden brown, about 30 minutes. Purée until smooth.

Nutrition Tip

The eyes have it. Carrots are the richest vegetable source of beta-carotene, which is converted to vitamin A in the liver. Your baby's developing vision relies on adequate amounts of this vitamin. The body preferentially uses vitamin A in specific areas of the eye giving your baby the ability to see well in the dark (night vision).

1½ cups	coarsely chopped peeled carrots	375 mL
1 cup	cold water	250 mL

1. In a saucepan, combine carrots and water. Bring to a boil over medium heat. Reduce heat to low and simmer until carrots are very soft, about 25 minutes.

2. Transfer to a blender or use an immersion blender in the saucepan. Purée until smooth. Let cool until warm to the touch or transfer to an airtight container and refrigerate for up to 3 days or freeze for up to 1 month.

Nutrients per serving (¼ cup/50 mL)

Calories 20	Dietary fiber . . . . . . 1.3 g
Protein . . . . 0.5 g	Sodium . . . . 34.9 mg
Total fat . . . . 0.1 g	Calcium . . . . 17.6 mg
Saturated fat. . . . . . 0.0 g	Iron . . . . 0.1 mg
Carbohydrates. . . . . 4.6 g	Vitamin C. . . . . . . 2.8 mg

Not just for babies

For the greatest carrot ginger soup EVER, follow the instructions for roasted carrots (see Chef Jordan's Tips), double the quantity and add ½ cup (125 mL) unsweetened coconut milk and 2 tbsp (25 mL) fresh gingerroot while blending.

Sweet Pea Purée

This vibrant green purée will be one of your baby's favorites. It looks great and tastes even better!

**Makes about
1¼ cups (300 mL)**

■ ■ ■

Chef Jordan's Tips

Generally speaking, peas in the pod can be difficult to find and, when available, are very expensive! Individually frozen peas, preferably organic, packed at their peak of freshness, are available in most grocery stores. They make a great alternative to fresh.

Nutrition Tip

Peas provide a great source of complex carbohydrates, which are slowly broken down into glucose (a simple sugar) by the digestive system. Since the brain relies entirely on glucose to function, complex carbohydrates provide the perfect fuel to optimize your baby's physical and mental activities.

| 1¼ cups | frozen sweet peas | 300 mL |
| 1¼ cups | water | 300 mL |

1. In a saucepan, combine peas and water. Bring to a boil over medium heat. Reduce heat to low and simmer until peas are soft, about 15 minutes. Let cool until warm to the touch.

2. Transfer to a blender or use an immersion blender in the saucepan. Purée until smooth. Serve immediately or transfer to an airtight container and refrigerate for up to 3 days or freeze for up to 1 month.

Nutrients per serving (¼ cup/50 mL)	
Calories 23	Dietary fiber . . . . . . 1.5 g
Protein . . . . 1.5 g	Sodium . . . . 78.7 mg
Total fat . . . . 0.0 g	Calcium . . . . 1.8 mg
Saturated fat. . . . . . 0.0 g	Iron . . . . 0.4 mg
Carbohydrates. . . . . 4.6 g	Vitamin C. . . . . . . 2.3 mg

Not just for babies

After puréeing, spoon off dinner for your baby and add ½ cup (125 mL) of chicken stock and 2 leaves of mint. Purée again. You'll have an excellent sauce to serve with grilled salmon fillets.

Roasted Beet Purée

I always thought beets were a rather bland vegetable, and then I roasted them whole. Now this is one of my favorite flavors.

Makes about 1½ cups (375 mL)

■ ■ ■

Chef Jordan's Tips

Before roasting, scrub beets with a soft brush under cool running water to remove all dirt and grit. Pat dry.

The easiest way to peel beets after roasting is to cool them overnight; the skins will come off without a struggle.

Nutrition Tip

Even at this tender young age your baby's liver has more than 500 functions. One is to keep her blood clean by filtering out both internal and external toxins. Beets have a stimulating effect on the liver and its detoxification processes. Just don't be alarmed if your baby's bowel movements and urine are dyed red after enjoying this purée. Beets contain anthocyanin, a powerful antioxidant that stimulates this condition, known as beeturia.

• **Preheat oven to 350°F (180°C)**

| 1½ lbs | fresh beets (3 large) | 750 g |
| 1 cup | water | 250 mL |

1. On a baking sheet, roast beets in a preheated oven until fork tender, about 2½ hours. Let cool for at least 3 hours (see Tips, left).
2. Peel beets, roughly chop and transfer to a saucepan with water. Bring to a boil over medium heat.
3. Transfer to a blender or use an immersion blender in the saucepan. Purée until smooth. Let cool until warm to the touch or transfer to an airtight container and refrigerate for up to 3 days or freeze for up to 1 month.

Nutrients per serving (¼ cup/50 mL)			
Calories	54	Dietary fiber	3.5 g
Protein	2.0 g	Sodium	98.8 mg
Total fat	0.2 g	Calcium	21.3 mg
Saturated fat	0.0 g	Iron	1.0 mg
Carbohydrates	12.0 g	Vitamin C	6.1 mg

Not just for babies

Combine ½ cup (125 mL) roasted beet purée with ¼ cup (50 mL) extra virgin olive oil and 1 tbsp (15 mL) of your favorite vinegar. Serve over a goat cheese salad.

Caramelized Parsnip Purée

When I was growing up, my mother rarely cooked parsnips. I learned about this very sweet tuber in culinary school. Roasting creates a candy-like purée. What's not to love?

Makes about 2 cups (500 mL)

▪ ▪ ▪

Chef Jordan's Tips

When roasting vegetables, especially those containing a lot of sugar, drippings develop that adhere to the bottom of the cooking vessel. In professional kitchens this is called the *fond* and it is loaded with flavor that you don't want to lose. You can easily scrape the fond into the liquid using a rubber spatula or wooden spoon.

Nutrition Tip

Parsnips look like a white carrot but do not pale in the nutrients they contain. They are a good source of fiber, which helps to keep your baby's bowel healthy, and B vitamins that are used to produce energy and keep his metabolism humming. As a sweet, soft food, parsnips are another root vegetable that work well as an introductory food.

• **Preheat oven to 350°F (180°C)**

| 4 | parsnips, peeled and halved | 4 |
| 1½ cups | water | 375 mL |

1. On a baking sheet, roast parsnips in preheated oven until soft and golden brown, about 1 hour.
2. Chop parsnips and transfer to a saucepan with water. Bring to a boil over medium heat. Reduce heat to low and simmer until water is reduced by about half, about 5 minutes. Transfer to a blender or use an immersion blender in the saucepan. Purée until smooth. Let cool until warm to the touch or transfer to an airtight container and refrigerate for up to 3 days or freeze for up to 1 month.

Nutrients per serving (¼ cup/50 mL)

Calories	25	Dietary fiber	1.6 g
Protein	0.4 g	Sodium	4.7 mg
Total fat	0.1 g	Calcium	13.3 mg
Saturated fat	0.0 g	Iron	0.2 mg
Carbohydrates	6.0 g	Vitamin C	5.7 mg

Not just for babies

Make a big batch of these parsnips so Mom and Dad can enjoy them along with Baby, as a substitute for mashed potatoes.

Basic Quinoa

Some say it's a fruit. Others argue it's a seed. But there is no denying that this protein-packed pinhead-size "grain" is an ancient delicacy that is great for modern babies.

Makes about 1¼ cups (300 mL)

■ ■ ■

Chef Jordan's Tips

Depending upon where your baby is in terms of eating solid foods, quinoa can be puréed or left whole and added to another purée to provide a nutritional boost and textural contrast.

Toasting grains in a dry pan deepens their natural flavors.

Nutrition Tip

This ancient grain is gluten-free, has one of the highest iron contents of any grain and is a complete protein. That means it contains all eight essential amino acids, which are the building blocks of everything in your baby's body. We call them essential because they must be obtained from the diet. Most complete proteins are found in animal products, making quinoa a particularly valuable protein source for vegetarians.

½ cup	quinoa	125 mL
1 cup	water	250 mL

1. Warm a saucepan over medium heat. Add quinoa and toast, stirring constantly, until golden and fragrant, about 4 minutes.

2. Add water and bring to a boil. Cover, reduce heat to low and simmer for 15 minutes. Set aside to steep until quinoa is soft and water is absorbed, about 15 minutes. Let cool to room temperature before serving to Baby or transfer to an airtight container and refrigerate for up to 3 days.

Nutrients per serving (¼ cup/50 mL)

Calories 64	Dietary fiber . . . . . . 1.0 g
Protein . . . . 2.2 g	Sodium . . . . 5.0 mg
Total fat . . . . 1.0 g	Calcium . . . . 11.6 mg
Saturated fat. . . . . . 0.1 g	Iron . . . . 1.6 mg
Carbohydrates. . . . 11.7 g	Vitamin C. . . . . . . 0.0 mg

Not just for babies

Chill the quinoa after cooking and use it to make a cold salad with the addition of some chopped red or green onion, celery, carrots and vinaigrette. Or serve it warm with olive oil, fresh garlic and Parmesan cheese.

Simple Millet Cereal

I love the "nutty" flavor of millet. It is quite mild and aromatic, which your baby will love.

**Makes about
2 cups (500 mL)**

▪ ▪ ▪

Chef Jordan's Tips

Millet flour stores well
in an airtight container
in the refrigerator.

Nutrition Tip

Millet is a wonderful
grain for your baby. It
is gluten-free, easily
digestible and one of the
least allergenic grains.
It has a nice mild flavor
and a protein content
that is similar to wheat
and rice, so it will satisfy
a hungry baby's appetite.

3 cups	water	750 mL
¾ cup	millet flour (see page 51)	175 mL

1. In a saucepan, bring water to a boil over medium
   heat. Whisk millet flour into water and continue to
   cook, whisking often, until mixture is thick, about
   10 minutes. Remove from heat and let cool until
   warm to the touch. Serve immediately or transfer
   to an airtight container and refrigerate for up to
   3 days.

Nutrients per serving (¼ cup/50 mL)	
Calories 37	Dietary fiber . . . . . . 0.9 g
Protein . . . . 1.1 g	Sodium . . . . 2.7 mg
Total fat . . . . 0.4 g	Calcium . . . . 2.7 mg
Saturated fat . . . . . . 0.0 g	Iron . . . . 0.8 mg
Carbohydrates . . . . . 7.4 g	Vitamin C . . . . 0.0 mg

Not just for babies

The entire family can enjoy this cereal as a
morning porridge. Just add 2 tbsp (25 mL) maple
syrup and 1 tbsp (15 mL) brown sugar to every
1 cup (250 mL) of Simple Millet Cereal.

Brown Rice Cereal

The difference between making your own cereal and buying something from the grocery shelves is like the difference between night and day. Finding the 10 minutes it takes to make this recipe should be the biggest chore — it's really that easy.

Makes about 2¼ cups (550 mL)

■ ■ ■

Chef Jordan's Tips

You can purchase brown rice flour in natural food stores, but for me, it's all about ownership. I feel better about grinding my own flour rather than purchasing it in a bag. I get a certain pride from the work that goes into creating something for my children.

Nutrition Tip

Whole grains are an important component of any diet for many reasons (see page 55 for more on whole grains), not the least of which is their chromium content. Because chromium is found in the bran and the germ, a high percentage of this "ultra trace" mineral is lost when grains are refined. Chromium is responsible for regulating blood sugar, and a deficiency of this mineral is linked to the development of diabetes.

| 5 cups | water | 1.25 L |
| ¾ cup | brown rice flour (see page 51) | 175 mL |

1. In a saucepan, bring water to a boil over medium heat. Slowly whisk rice flour into water, stirring constantly to avoid clumping. Cook, whisking constantly, until liquid turns a chocolate brown and begins to thicken, about 10 minutes. Remove from heat and set aside for at least 1 hour (the mixture will become quite thick). Continue to whisk from time to time as it cools. Serve immediately or transfer to an airtight container and refrigerate for up to 3 days.

2. To serve, reheat ½ cup (125 mL) of cooked cereal with ¼ cup (50 mL) water in a saucepan over low heat just until warm.

Nutrients per serving (¼ cup/50 mL)	
Calories 48	Dietary fiber . . . . . . 0.6 g
Protein . . . . 1.0 g	Sodium . . . . 4.2 mg
Total fat . . . . 0.4 g	Calcium . . . . 4.6 mg
Saturated fat . . . . . . 0.1 g	Iron . . . . 0.3 mg
Carbohydrates . . . . 10.1 g	Vitamin C . . . . 0.0 mg

Not just for babies
Sorry folks, this really is just for babies.

Make Your Own Flour

From the Nutritionist

When you grind a whole grain, you are exposing the essential oils present in the germ of the grain. These oils are very beneficial to our bodies when they are fresh but can deteriorate quickly with exposure to oxygen, light and heat. Try to grind just enough flour for a day or two to preserve the freshness of these oils, and then store the unused portions in the fridge in an airtight glass container.

It takes just a few minutes to grind your own flour, and the results are worth every one of them because you produce the freshest, best-tasting flour there is. Some grains, such as millet and barley, benefit from a light toasting to bring out their natural flavor. To grind flour from harder grains such as barley and rice, we like to use a blender. For softer grains such as millet or oats, an immersion blender with a small cup attachment works just fine. A clean coffee grinder or spice grinder or a home flour mill also works well for all varieties of grains.

To make barley flour: In a saucepan over low heat, toast barley until aromatic, 3 to 5 minutes, stirring often to prevent burning. Remove from heat and set aside until completely cool. Transfer to a blender, in batches if necessary, and pulse until desired texture is achieved, about 4 minutes. Store in an airtight container in the refrigerator.

To make brown rice flour: Place long-grain brown rice in a blender, in batches if necessary, and pulse until desired consistency is achieved, about 3 minutes. (In a pinch, I use a combination of jasmine and short-grain brown rice.) Store in an airtight container in the refrigerator.

To make millet flour: In a saucepan over low heat, toast millet until aromatic, 3 to 5 minutes, stirring often to prevent burning. Remove from heat and set aside until completely cooled. Transfer to a blender (or an immersion blender with a small cup attachment), in batches if necessary, and pulse until desired texture is achieved, about 3 minutes. Store in an airtight container in the refrigerator.

To make oat flour: Place steel-cut (our preference for nutritional reasons) or rolled oats in a blender (or use an immersion blender with a small cup attachment), in batches if necessary, and pulse until desired consistency is achieved, about 2 minutes. Store in an airtight container in the refrigerator.

Simple Barley Cereal

Another way to introduce texture to your baby. If you're grinding barley rather than purchasing barley flour, grind some finely and leave the remainder a bit coarser to create textural contrast.

Makes about 2¼ cups (550 mL)

Chef Jordan's Tips

Homemade flours are quite easy to make and not at all time-consuming.

Nutrition Tip

There are three different ways of buying barley: hulled barley, pot barley and pearled barley. Pearled barley is the most refined because it has had most of the outer bran and germ layer removed. On the other end of the scale, hulled barley has only had the tough outer hull polished off and so it retains virtually all of its fiber and phytonutrients. Pot barley is somewhere in the middle. Flour made from hulled barley can be used in this recipe but be sure to double the cooking time to about 40 minutes, because this version has been tested using pearled barley.

3 cups	water	750 mL
¾ cup	barley flour (see page 51)	175 mL

1. In a saucepan, bring water to a boil over medium-low heat. Whisk flour into water and continue to cook, whisking often, until mixture is thick and flour is fully cooked, from 20 to 40 minutes (see Nutrition Tip, left). Remove from heat and let cool until warm to the touch. Serve immediately or transfer to an airtight container and refrigerate for up to 3 days.

Nutrients per serving (¼ cup/50 mL)

Calories	60	Dietary fiber	2.7 g
Protein	1.7 g	Sodium	3.7 mg
Total fat	0.3 g	Calcium	5.7 mg
Saturated fat	0.0 g	Iron	0.4 mg
Carbohydrates	13.0 g	Vitamin C	0.0 mg

Not just for babies

Sorry folks...this is just for babies!

Whole-Grain Oat Cereal with Grapes

I prefer this to the packaged instant oatmeal that people often use because it's convenient. It tastes better and it's healthier, too.

Makes about 3¼ cups (800 mL)

■ ■ ■

Chef Jordan's Tips
Grapes are easily substituted with puréed apples, pears, peaches, plums...you name it.

Nutrition Tip
Whole-grain oats are a rich source of fiber and phytonutrients and they provide long-lasting energy for your baby. Typically people following a gluten-free diet have been advised to stay away from oats, but recent studies show that oats do not appear to contain gluten. Rather, it is the cross-contamination that occurs during harvesting, milling and processing that may cause problems. If you are following a gluten-free diet, you may be able to include oats in your diet, but be sure to purchase them from a source that guarantees they are gluten-free.

3 cups	water	750 mL
¾ cup	oat flour (see page 51)	175 mL
¼ cup	red or green grapes, seeded, if necessary, and puréed	50 mL

1. In a saucepan, bring water to a boil over medium heat. Whisk oat flour into water and continue to cook, whisking constantly, until mixture is thick, about 5 minutes. Add puréed grapes and whisk thoroughly to incorporate. Remove from heat and let cool until warm to the touch. Serve immediately or transfer to an airtight container and refrigerate for up to 3 days.

Nutrients per serving (¼ cup/50 mL)

Calories 35	Dietary fiber . . . . . . 1.0 g
Protein . . . . 1.4 g	Sodium . . . . 1.6 mg
Total fat . . . . 0.6 g	Calcium . . . . 6.8 mg
Saturated fat. . . . . . 0.1 g	Iron . . . . 0.4 mg
Carbohydrates. . . . . 6.9 g	Vitamin C. . . . . . . 0.4 mg

Not just for babies
You can add diced apples and fresh cinnamon or even dried apricots and a dash of maple syrup to this cereal. There are many great combinations...you should try every single one of them.

Quinoa and Banana Purée

This is a great recipe to introduce quinoa to your baby. The sweetness of the bananas makes it a pleasure to eat.

Makes about 1¼ cups (300 mL)

1	banana, peeled	1
1 cup	water	250 mL
½ cup	cooked quinoa (see recipe, page 48)	125 mL

1. In a saucepan, combine bananas, water and quinoa. Bring to a boil over medium heat. Reduce heat to low and simmer until bananas are soft, about 5 minutes.

2. Transfer to a blender or use an immersion blender in the saucepan. Purée until smooth. Let cool until warm to the touch. Serve immediately or transfer to an airtight container and refrigerate for up to 3 days.

Chef Jordan's Tips

When choosing bananas for cooking, I tend to use the most ripe. I'll choose from any of the sweet bananas available. Regular yellow long bananas, dwarf, finger or red bananas all work well for baby food purées. The only variety I recommend avoiding is the plantain. While there are many delicious plantain recipes, puréeing them for baby food is not an appropriate use. Plantains are less sweet and starchier than their cousins, and should never be eaten raw.

Nutrition Tip

Bananas have a low allergenic potential and quinoa is gluten-free. Consequently, this is a relatively safe recipe to try if you think your baby might have an allergic reaction, based on allergies you or your partner may have.

Nutrients per serving (¼ cup/50 mL)	
Calories 46	Dietary fiber ...... 1.0 g
Protein .... 1.2 g	Sodium .... 3.7 mg
Total fat .... 0.5 g	Calcium .... 7.8 mg
Saturated fat...... 0.1 g	Iron .... 0.7 mg
Carbohydrates.... 10.1 g	Vitamin C....... 2.1 mg

Not just for babies

Turn this into a salsa by adding 1 tbsp (15 mL) each unsweetened coconut milk and diced tropical fruit. Serve with fish, such as grilled red snapper.

Wholesome Whole Grains

All grains start out as whole grains. They have three distinct parts — the endosperm (which contains the starch), the bran (where the fiber is) and the germ (which houses many of the good fats). When a grain is processed, it loses some or all of the bran and germ, leaving only the endosperm, the least nutritious part of the grain. Polished white rice, for instance, has had all of its bran and germ removed, leaving only the starch component.

It is well known that the high fiber content of whole grains promotes digestive health, but newer studies are suggesting a wide range of benefits associated with whole-grain consumption. Studies show that regular consumption of whole grains reduces the risk of heart disease, some types of cancer, stroke and type-2 diabetes. People who eat whole grains regularly have a healthier waist-to-hip ratio and lower blood serum cholesterol. Whole grains have been found to contain valuable antioxidants as well as a range of B vitamins, vitamin E, magnesium and iron. Be sure to include whole grains daily in your baby's diet to maximize these health benefits.

Apple and Fig Brown Rice Cereal

Figs add a superb, unique sweetness to the rather bland canvas provided by brown rice!

Makes about 3 cups (750 mL)

◼ ◼ ◼

Chef Jordan's Tips

Fresh figs are often available but I also love the dried versions. Like most dried fruits, they are much sweeter and have a much more pronounced flavor than their fresh counterparts.

Nutrition Tip

Figs are entirely under-rated as a super food for babies. They are a tremendous source of fiber and minerals, such as potassium, magnesium, calcium and iron. They are also a good energy food, support blood formation and are helpful for relieving constipation.

Buy organic apples

5 cups	water	1.25 L
¾ cup	brown rice flour (see page 51)	175 mL
2 cups	diced cored peeled apples (about 2 medium apples)	500 mL
½ cup	chopped dried figs	125 mL

1. In a saucepan, bring water to a boil over medium heat. Slowly whisk rice flour into water, stirring constantly to avoid clumping. Cook, whisking constantly, until liquid turns a chocolate brown and begins to thicken, about 10 minutes. Add apples and figs and stir well to combine. Remove from heat and set aside for at least 1 hour or for up to 2 hours, whisking from time to time. The mixture will become quite thick as it cools. Serve immediately or transfer to an airtight container and refrigerate for up to 3 days.

2. To serve the cereal, combine with water in a ratio of ½ cup (125 mL) cooked cereal to ¼ cup (50 mL) water. Warm in a saucepan over low heat.

Nutrients per serving (¼ cup/50 mL)	
Calories 67	Dietary fiber . . . . . . 1.8 g
Protein . . . . 1.0 g	Sodium . . . . 4.8 mg
Total fat . . . . 0.4 g	Calcium . . . . 18.7 mg
Saturated fat. . . . . . 0.1 g	Iron . . . . 0.4 mg
Carbohydrates. . . . 15.7 g	Vitamin C. . . . . . . 1.1 mg

Not just for babies
Sorry folks. This one is too much of a stretch for adults.

Tofu, Bosc Pears and Banana

This sweet purée is a great way to introduce tofu to your baby. Tofu is one of those "white canvas" foods that combines easily with other ingredients, such as fruits and vegetables.

**Makes about
1 cup (250 mL)**

■ ■ ■

Chef Jordan's Tips

In season, I prefer to use Bosc pears in this recipe because they have a slightly tart flavor, which nicely counters the sweetness of the cooked bananas, creating an excellent balance of flavors. If they aren't available, use an equal quantity of Anjou or Bartlett pears.

Nutrition Tip

Tofu is a complete protein from a nonanimal source. It is also a source of iron, which is used for transporting oxygen throughout the body. Your baby's iron stores will begin to decline at about the six-month mark, making iron from the diet a key nutritional consideration. Vegetable sources of iron are better absorbed when eaten with vitamin C, which in this recipe is provided by the pears.

Buy organic pears

¾ cup	water	175 mL
½ cup	chopped cored Bosc pear (see Tips, left)	125 mL
½	banana	½
¼ cup	diced firm tofu	50 mL

1. In a saucepan, combine water, pear and banana. Bring to a boil over medium heat. Reduce heat to low and simmer until pear is fork tender and water has reduced by about one-quarter, about 5 minutes. Remove from heat and add tofu.

2. Transfer to a blender or use an immersion blender in the saucepan. Purée until smooth. Let cool until warm to the touch or transfer to an airtight container and refrigerate for up to 3 days or freeze for up to 1 month.

Nutrients per serving (¼ cup/50 mL)	
Calories 26	Dietary fiber . . . . . . 1.0 g
Protein . . . . 0.4 g	Sodium . . . . 1.7 mg
Total fat . . . . 0.2 g	Calcium . . . . 6.8 mg
Saturated fat. . . . . . 0.0 g	Iron . . . . 0.1 mg
Carbohydrates. . . . . 6.6 g	Vitamin C. . . . . . . 2.2 mg

Not just for babies

I recently met Tamar and a few friends for a quick lunch at a hot new breakfast restaurant and had a soy milk shake with banana and pears that reminded me of this recipe. It would be equally good (or even better) if you used this purée as the base and added strawberry ice cream. Put your child down for a nap and enjoy it as a treat during a rare five minutes of peace and quiet.

Roasted Apple, Blueberry and Pear

Blueberries add a jelly-like consistency to purées. The flavor and texture of this one is appealingly unique.

Makes about 3 cups (750 mL)

■ ■ ■

Chef Jordan's Tips

I prefer to use fresh berries, but frozen berries are readily available and a good option when fresh are not in season.

If you have access to wild blueberries, which have a unique flavor, use them in this recipe.

Nutrition Tip

This dynamic trio of apple, blueberry and pear is a potent source of vitamin C. The effects of this antioxidant go well beyond helping with the common cold. Vitamin C is crucial in the formation and maintenance of collagen. As the foundation of connective tissue found in skin, bones, joints and ligaments, collagen gives support and shape to your baby's body.

Buy organic apples and pears

• Preheat oven to 350°F (180°C)

3 cups	chopped cored apples (about 3)	750 mL
2¼ cups	finely chopped cored pears (about 3)	550 mL
1 cup	water	250 mL
½ cup	blueberries	125 mL

1. In an ovenproof skillet, roast apples in preheated oven until skins are golden brown, about 40 minutes. Transfer skillet to the stove-top.

2. Add pears, water and blueberries. Bring to a boil over medium heat. Reduce heat and simmer, stirring occasionally until pears are tender, about 10 minutes.

3. Transfer to a blender or a bowl and use an immersion blender. Purée until smooth. Let cool until warm to the touch or transfer to an airtight container and refrigerate for up to 3 days or freeze for up to 1 month.

Nutrients per serving (¼ cup/50 mL)	
Calories 39	Dietary fiber . . . . . . 1.9 g
Protein . . . . 0.3 g	Sodium . . . . 1.3 mg
Total fat . . . . 0.1 g	Calcium . . . . 5.8 mg
Saturated fat. . . . . . 0.0 g	Iron . . . . 0.1 mg
Carbohydrates. . . . 10.4 g	Vitamin C. . . . . . . 3.5 mg

Not just for babies

In your blender, combine 1 cup (250 mL) purée with 1 cup (250 mL) full-fat yogurt to make a great smoothie for you and the family.

Nectarine and Carrot Purée

A grand recipe when nectarines are in season!

**Makes about
1¾ cups (425 mL)**

■ ■ ■

Chef Jordan's Tips
Substitute peaches for the nectarines.

In the absence of seasonal nectarines or peaches, use dried fruit. Dried fruit can be much sweeter than fresh because the sugars are concentrated, so the flavor of your purée won't be compromised by their use. In this recipe, use 1 cup (250 mL) of dried fruit in place of the fresh.

Nutrition Tip
Nectarines and carrots both contain significant amounts of natural sugars that your baby uses as fuel for her constantly active body. Don't be afraid of trying carrots, or any vegetable, as a morning purée.

Buy organic nectarines

2½ cups	quartered nectarines (about 3)	625 mL
1¼ cups	coarsely chopped peeled carrots	300 mL
1 cup	water	250 mL

1. In a saucepan, combine nectarines, carrots and water. Bring to a boil over medium heat. Reduce heat to low and simmer until carrots are fork tender and most of the liquid has evaporated, about 30 minutes. Let cool to room temperature.

2. Transfer to a blender or use an immersion blender in the saucepan. Purée until smooth. Let cool until warm to the touch or transfer to an airtight container and refrigerate for up to 3 days or freeze for up to 1 month.

Nutrients per serving (¼ cup/50 mL)	
Calories 31	Dietary fiber . . . . . . 1.5 g
Protein . . . . 0.7 g	Sodium . . . . 16.8 mg
Total fat . . . . 0.2 g	Calcium . . . . 11.5 mg
Saturated fat. . . . . . 0.0 g	Iron . . . . 0.2 mg
Carbohydrates. . . . . 7.4 g	Vitamin C. . . . . . . 4.0 mg

Not just for babies
For a delicious and healthy summer snack make a "mousse" by folding in a touch of honey and vanilla yogurt to some of the purée.

Apricot Acorn Squash Purée

If your baby is going to wear her food, this is a great color.

**Makes about
2 cups (500 mL)**

■ ■ ■

Chef Jordan's Tips
The recommended cooking time is accurate if the acorn squash is cut to the same size as the apricots. If not, be sure to cook long enough for the squash to become fork tender.

Dried apricots can be used in place of the fresh. Substitute 3 dried apricots for the fresh.

Nutrition Tip
The combination of apricot and acorn squash makes this recipe a heavy hitter for the antioxidant beta-carotene. It also provides a number of important minerals for infants, including calcium, iron, magnesium, phosphorus and potassium.

2 cups	coarsely chopped peeled acorn squash (10 oz/300 g)	500 mL
6	apricots, pitted (about 8 oz/250 g)	6
1 cup	water	250 mL

1. In a saucepan, combine squash, apricots and water. Bring to a boil over medium heat. Reduce heat to low and simmer until squash is fork tender, about 20 minutes.

2. Transfer to a blender or use an immersion blender in the saucepan. Purée until smooth. Let cool until warm to the touch or transfer to an airtight container and refrigerate for up to 3 days or freeze for up to 1 month.

Nutrients per serving (1/4 cup/50 mL)	
Calories 30	Dietary fiber . . . . . . 1.2 g
Protein . . . . 0.7 g	Sodium . . . . 2.3 mg
Total fat . . . . 0.2 g	Calcium . . . . 17.3 mg
Saturated fat. . . . . . 0.0 g	Iron . . . . 0.4 mg
Carbohydrates. . . . . 7.4 g	Vitamin C. . . . . . . 7.3 mg

Not just for babies
While testing recipes for this book, I often experimented with flavor pairings based on what Tamar and I were having for dinner. One evening, we happened to have a pistachio crusted double-thick pork chop (if you're thinking Tamar is a lucky woman, I would agree), which we tried with this purée. It was, as the saying goes, "a match made in heaven." The fresh flavors of the apricots and squash stood out from the pork chop while simultaneously complementing it.

Green Bean Purée with Fresh Basil

"We all eat with our eyes first"...that is why a vibrant green color is so important. It will ensure your kids will WANT to eat these vegetables (see Tips, below).

Makes about 1 cup (250 mL)

■ ■ ■

Chef Jordan's Tips

The best way to achieve a vibrant green for vegetables, in the absence of salt, is to keep the water at a rolling boil. When cooking larger quantities, cook in batches, being careful not to overload the water, which will lower the temperature.

Be sure to use fresh basil. In my opinion, basil is one herb that doesn't maintain its flavor when dried.

Nutrition Tip

There is more to basil than meets the nose. This fragrant herb has long been used to help relieve stomach cramps, vomiting and constipation. It is packed with nutrients such as antioxidants, acts as an immune stimulant and also has antibacterial properties.

1 cup	water	250 mL
1½ cups	green beans, trimmed	375 mL
1 tsp	chopped fresh basil (see Tips, left)	5 mL
	Ice cubes	

1. In a saucepan, bring water to a rolling boil over high heat. Add green beans. Cover, maintaining a rolling boil, and boil until beans are soft, about 10 minutes.

2. Add basil. Transfer to a blender or use an immersion blender in the saucepan. Purée until smooth. Pour mixture into a bowl and place over top of another bowl filled with ice. Stir often to stop the cooking process and ensure that the beans maintain their beautiful green color. Serve when warm to the touch or transfer to an airtight container and refrigerate for up to 3 days or freeze for up to 1 month.

Nutrients per serving (¼ cup/50 mL)

Calories	10	Dietary fiber	1.5 g
Protein	0.5 g	Sodium	1.8 mg
Total fat	0.0 g	Calcium	22.1 mg
Saturated fat	0.0 g	Iron	0.2 mg
Carbohydrates	2.5 g	Vitamin C	3.0 mg

Not just for babies

Try folding the purée into your mashed potatoes for a variation on the "same old thing." Combine the purée with milk or cream and butter and bring to a simmer over low heat. Transfer to hot mashed potatoes and stir to combine.

Honeydew, Blueberry and Mint Purée

This recipe is so refreshing! Every summer, at the cottage, I turn it into ice pops for my nephew Josh and my son, Jonah, which they love. They are a cinch to make, frozen in ice cube trays with regular Popsicle sticks.

Makes about 6 cups (1.5 L)

5 cups	coarsely chopped seeded peeled honeydew melon (about 1 large)	1.25 L
¾ cup	blueberries	175 mL
½	cup water	125 mL
3	mint leaves, chopped	3

1. In a saucepan, combine melon, blueberries and water. Bring to a boil over medium heat. (You just want to "marry" the flavors without affecting the texture of the melon.)

2. Transfer to a blender or use an immersion blender in the saucepan. Add mint and purée until fully incorporated, about 1 minute. Let cool until warm to the touch (see Tips, left) or transfer to an airtight container and refrigerate for up to 3 days or freeze for up to 1 month.

Chef Jordan's Tips

My preference is to serve this purée cold, right from the refrigerator. I prefer the flavor of honeydew melon when it is cold.

Although mint is a wonderful addition to this purée, I recommend using herbs from your garden, if available. An equal quantity of thyme, sage or oregano would work beautifully with these flavors.

Nutrition Tip

Mint is very tummy friendly. Its natural oils help relax the smooth muscle of the intestines, which may help relieve spasms and gas. If your baby has been struggling with gas during the day, this recipe may be a good choice to make in the evening to reduce discomfort and help her sleep.

Nutrients per serving (¼ cup/50 mL)	
Calories 3	Dietary fiber . . . . . . 0.1 g
Protein . . . . 0.0 g	Sodium . . . . 0.2 mg
Total fat . . . . 0.0 g	Calcium . . . . 0.4 mg
Saturated fat. . . . . 0.0 g	Iron . . . . 0.5 mg
Carbohydrates. . . . . 0.7 g	Vitamin C. . . . . . . 0.4 mg

Not just for babies

This purée makes an excellent cold soup, which is a great way to cool down on a summer day. Add ½ cup (125 mL) of freshly squeezed orange juice to every 1 cup (250 mL) of purée.

Plum and Blueberry Purée

When my son, Jonah, was in this age bracket he loved this purée with his hot cereal in the morning. Try this with the millet (see page 49) or brown rice cereal (see page 50) recipes. You and your children will love the combination!

Makes about 2 cups (500 mL)

■ ■ ■

Chef Jordan's Tips
Add 1 tsp (5 mL) of agave nectar or honey to this superb purée and transform it into wonderful jam-like spread to put on your French toast in the morning. Be sure not to serve it to a baby who is younger than a year, because honey contains toxins that may be harmful.

Nutrition Tip
It's well known that cranberries help promote urinary tract health. But so do blueberries! In fact they contain proanthocyanidins, the same compounds that decrease the ability of offending bacteria to stick to the lining of the bladder. Because the bacteria can't stick, they are flushed out with the urine, helping to prevent urinary tract infections, which are very common in the first year of life.

1½ cups	sliced pitted plums (about 3 medium-size plums)	375 mL
1 cup	blueberries	250 mL
½ cup	water	125 mL

1. In a saucepan, combine plums, blueberries and water. Bring to a boil over medium heat. Reduce heat to low and simmer until plums are soft, about 5 minutes.

2. In a colander set over a bowl, strain fruit, reserving cooking liquid. Transfer fruit to a blender or return to saucepan and use an immersion blender. Purée until smooth, adding enough of the reserved liquid to attain desired consistency. Let cool until warm to the touch or transfer to an airtight container and refrigerate for up to 3 days or freeze for up to 1 month.

Nutrients per serving (¼ cup/50 mL)	
Calories 32	Dietary fiber . . . . . . 1.2 g
Protein . . . . 0.5 g	Sodium . . . . 0.8 mg
Total fat . . . . 0.2 g	Calcium . . . . 4.2 mg
Saturated fat. . . . . . 0.0 g	Iron . . . . 0.1 mg
Carbohydrates. . . . . 8.1 g	Vitamin C. . . . . . . 6.0 mg

Not just for babies
Tamar and I are self-proclaimed cheese freaks, my favorite being semisoft goat cheeses. The flavor combination of this sweet yet tart purée combined with goat cheese is astounding. Simply spread a small bit onto flat bread, a cracker or sliced bread, lather the cheese on top and enjoy. Soft goat cheeses are readily available at supermarkets.

Zucchini and Basil Purée

I will always remember the first time I tried this flavor combination. It was a Friday night special at Pascal restaurant in Newport Beach, Calif. My cook, Katia, created a flan for an appetizer using this exact purée. It was a taste I've always remembered.

Makes about 1¼ cups (300 mL)

■ ■ ■

Chef Jordan's Tips
If zucchini isn't available, substitute an equal quantity of another summer squash such as crook-neck squash, yellow zucchini or pattypan squash (my personal favorite).

Nutrition Tip
Keeping your baby well hydrated is vital. Zucchini, which is 95 per cent water, is a good food source of water for your baby. Zucchini is also a source of folic acid, or folate, which your baby needs for energy and to create red and white blood cells and keep them functioning. Folate plays an integral role in keeping the blueprint of your baby's cell structure (DNA) forming correctly.

2¼ cups	coarsely chopped zucchini (about 3 small)	550 mL
1/2 cup	water	125 mL
3	basil leaves	3

1. In a saucepan, combine zucchini and water. Bring to a boil over medium heat. Cook until zucchini is soft and most of the liquid is absorbed, about 10 minutes. Let cool to room temperature.

2. Add basil. Transfer to a blender or use an immersion blender in the saucepan. Purée until smooth. Let cool until warm to the touch or transfer to an airtight container and refrigerate for up to 3 days or freeze for up to 1 month.

Nutrients per serving (¼ cup/50 mL)

Calories	8	Dietary fiber	0.6 g
Protein	0.6 g	Sodium	5.8 mg
Total fat	0.1 g	Calcium	8.8 mg
Saturated fat	0.0 g	Iron	0.2 mg
Carbohydrates	1.7 g	Vitamin C	8.7 mg

Not just for babies
After spooning off a portion for Baby, turn this into a casserole by adding 1 cup (250 mL) diced raw zucchini, 1 cup (250 mL) fresh chopped tomatoes, 1/2 cup (125 mL) bread crumbs and 1/2 cup (125 mL) grated Parmesan cheese to the remainder. Transfer to a small casserole dish and sprinkle with 1 tbsp (15 mL) Parmesan cheese. Bake in a preheated oven (300°F/150°C) until golden brown on top and warm throughout, about 25 minutes.

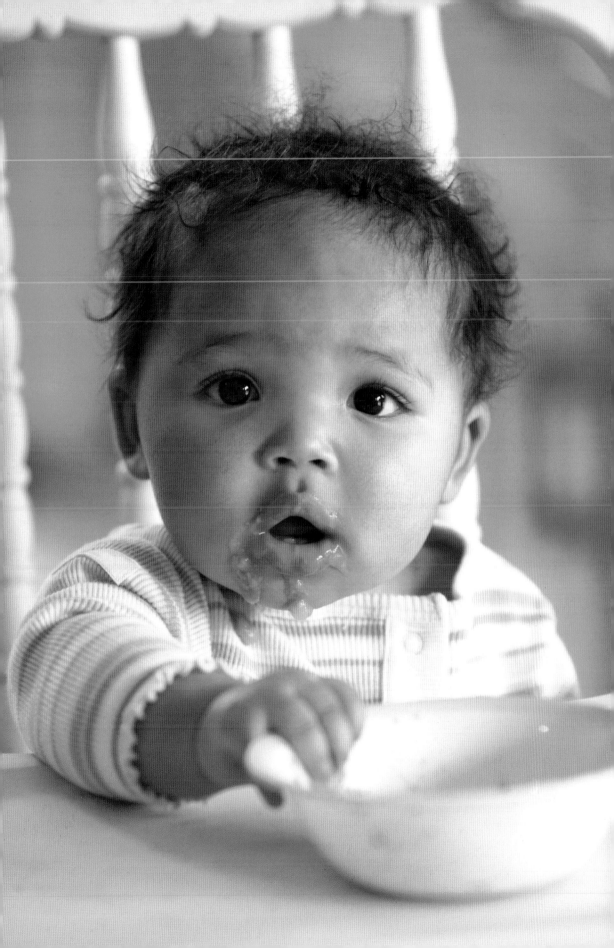

Mango Purée (page 39), Broccoli Purée (page 40),
Roasted Sweet Potato Purée (page 42) and Roasted Beet Purée (page 46)

Potato, Parsnip and Chicken Soup with
Chive Parsley "Pistou" (page 98)

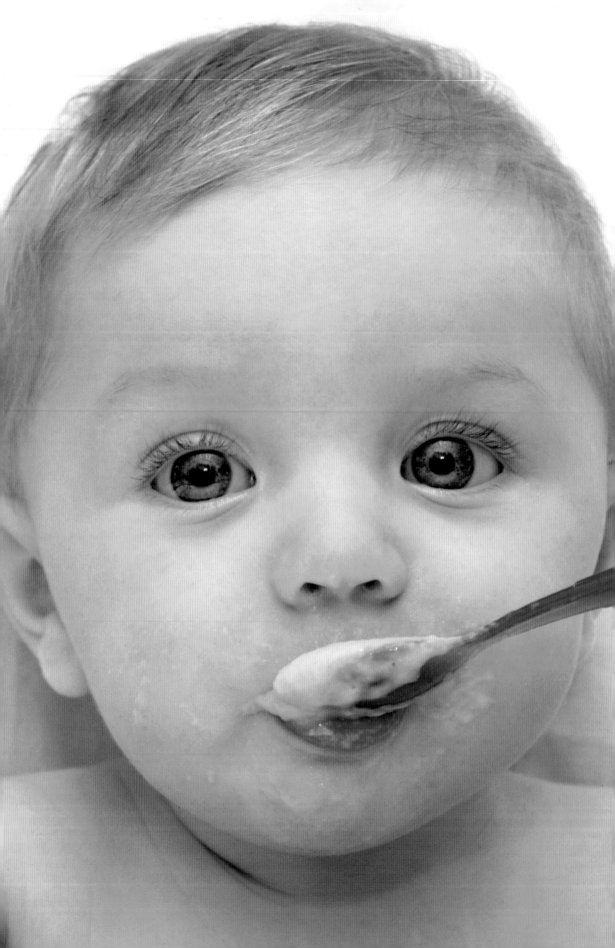

Cauliflower and Parsnip Purée

This is a wonderfully sweet purée your child will love!

**Makes about
2 cups (500 mL)**

■ ■ ■

Chef Jordan's Tips
Always take care when adding hot liquids to a blender. Fill the container no more than half full or allow to cool before blending.

Nutrition Tip
Your baby's bones are active and dynamic living things. Cauliflower contains a significant amount of vitamin K, which is vital for building and maintaining strong bones, among other benefits. This vitamin activates a protein that anchors calcium inside the bones. Other sources of vitamin K include broccoli, cabbage and leafy greens such as spinach.

2 cups	water	500 mL
2 cups	cauliflower florets	500 mL
½ cup	chopped peeled parsnip	125 mL

1. In a saucepan, combine water, cauliflower and parsnip. Bring to a boil over medium heat. Reduce heat to low and simmer until cauliflower and parsnip are fork tender, about 20 minutes. In a colander set over a bowl, drain vegetables, reserving cooking liquid.

2. Transfer vegetables to a blender or return to saucepan and use an immersion blender. Purée until smooth, adding reserved cooking liquid, if necessary, to achieve desired consistency. Let cool until warm to the touch or transfer to an airtight container and refrigerate for up to 3 days or freeze for up to 1 month.

Nutrients per serving (¼ cup/50 mL)	
Calories 9	Dietary fiber . . . . . . 0.7 g
Protein . . . . 0.3 g	Sodium . . . . 8.2 mg
Total fat . . . . 0.0 g	Calcium . . . . 9.4 mg
Saturated fat. . . . . . 0.0 g	Iron . . . . 0.1 mg
Carbohydrates. . . . . 2.2 g	Vitamin C. . . . . . . 7.2 mg

Not just for babies
This purée is superb with fish, either a whole roasted fish or a simple grilled fillet.

Cauliflower and Chickpea Chowder

This hearty purée is wonderful for dinner for the whole family especially on cold winter days. You can make a big batch just by doubling or tripling the recipe.

Makes about 2 cups (500 mL)

■ ■ ■

Chef Jordan's Tips

When making this recipe you can soak and cook your own dried chickpeas or use a brand of organically grown canned chickpeas with no salt added.

Nutrition Tip

Chickpeas (also known as garbanzo beans) are very high in fiber and are a complex carbohydrate. They are slowly broken down by the digestive system, providing sustained energy and balanced blood sugar levels. This purée will fill your baby's tummy and keep him satiated. It's a great dish to take along when the family is on the road and the time between feedings may be slightly longer than usual.

1²⁄₃ cups	drained, rinsed cooked chickpeas (see page 77)	400 mL
1²⁄₃ cups	water	400 mL
¹⁄₃ cup	cauliflower florets	75 mL
2	mint leaves	2

1. In a saucepan, combine chickpeas, water and cauliflower. Bring to a boil over medium heat. Reduce heat to low and simmer until cauliflower is fork tender, about 25 minutes.

2. Add mint. Transfer to a blender or use an immersion blender in the saucepan. Purée until smooth. Let cool until warm to the touch or transfer to an airtight container and refrigerate for up to 3 days or freeze for up to 1 month.

Nutrients per serving (¹⁄₄ cup/50 mL)	
Calories 57	Dietary fiber . . . . . . 2.7 g
Protein . . . . 3.1 g	Sodium . . . . 4.9 mg
Total fat . . . . 0.9 g	Calcium . . . . 19.0 mg
Saturated fat . . . . . . 0.1 g	Iron . . . . 1.0 mg
Carbohydrates . . . . . 9.6 g	Vitamin C . . . . 2.0 mg

Not just for babies

This purée makes a great dip for chips or cut-up vegetables. Add 1 tbsp (15 mL) chopped chives and ¹⁄₃ cup (75 mL) full-fat sour cream to ¹⁄₂ cup (125 mL) of purée — your family will love it!

Watermelon, Peach and Blueberry Purée

Your kids will love the fresh flavors of this purée.

Makes about 4 cups (1 L)

∎ ∎ ∎

Chef Jordan's Tips
Although seedless watermelons make your life easier when puréeing, the freshest local melons are the best, seedless or not. The best way to remove the seeds is with your best kitchen tools: your hands.

Nutrition Tip
The body needs enzymes as activators to kick start every metabolic function. This purée is completely uncooked, which preserves your baby's internal enzymes and offers added "spark plugs" naturally present in the fruits to aid in the full digestion and absorption of proteins, fats and carbohydrates.

Buy organic peaches

2¼ cups	chopped seedless watermelon (about 1½ lbs/750 g)	550 mL
2 cups	sliced pitted peaches (about 3)	500 mL
¼ cup	fresh or frozen blueberries	50 mL

1. In a blender, combine watermelon, peaches and blueberries. Purée until smooth. Serve immediately or transfer to an airtight container and refrigerate for up to 3 days or freeze for up to 1 month.

Nutrients per serving (¼ cup/50 mL)	
Calories 15	Dietary fiber . . . . . . 0.5 g
Protein . . . . 0.3 g	Sodium . . . . 0.7 mg
Total fat . . . . 0.1 g	Calcium . . . . 2.8 mg
Saturated fat. . . . . . 0.0 g	Iron . . . . 0.1 mg
Carbohydrates. . . . . 4.3 g	Vitamin C. . . . . . . 2.7 mg

Not just for babies
With the addition of crushed ice, orange juice and fresh berries, this makes an excellent summer punch for you and your adult guests.

Avocado, Carrot and Cucumber Purée

This recipe, which uses raw ingredients, is very refreshing. Consider it an infant gazpacho minus the tomatoes.

Makes about 1¾ cups (425 mL)

▪ ▪ ▪

Chef Jordan's Tips

Avocados tend to oxidize (turn brown) quickly. One trick, in the absence of lemon juice, which we don't suggest introducing to your baby until after 12 months, is to combine all the ingredients before peeling the avocado. This gives you something to mix with the avocado, delaying the onset of oxidization. For storage, make sure the plastic wrap directly touches the purée to prevent oxygen from reaching the mixture.

Nutrition Tip

This raw recipe is chock-full of enzymes, which help your baby digest and absorb her food. Adding cucumber to your baby's diet helps to keep her hydrated while providing vitamins A and C, along with folate.

¾ cup	chopped pitted peeled avocado (see Tips, left)	175 mL
½ cup	chopped seeded peeled English cucumber	125 mL
¼ cup	grated peeled carrot	50 mL
¼ cup	water	50 mL
3	mint leaves	3

1. In a blender, combine avocado, cucumber, carrot, water and mint. Purée until smooth. Serve immediately or transfer to an airtight container and refrigerate for up to 3 days (see Tips, left).

Nutrients per serving (¼ cup/50 mL)

Calories	27	Dietary fiber	1.2 g
Protein	0.4 g	Sodium	3.8 mg
Total fat	2.3 g	Calcium	4.6 mg
Saturated fat	0.3 g	Iron	0.1 mg
Carbohydrates	1.8 g	Vitamin C	2.1 mg

Not just for babies

This is an excellent dip for crudités. Scoop off some for your baby and add 2 tbsp (25 mL) freshly squeezed lemon juice, a dash of kosher salt and freshly ground black pepper before serving with cut-up vegetables of your choice.

Red Lentil and Apple

This is an excellent recipe to introduce lentils to your baby, because he will be familiar with the flavor of apples, ensuring a comfort level with the foreign texture of lentils.

Makes about 3 cups (750 mL)

▪ ▪ ▪

Chef Jordan's Tips

If you require more water for cooking the lentils, make sure it's hot before adding it to the pan so you won't lower the temperature and slow the cooking.

Nutrition Tip

Steaming or boiling pulls some nutrients from food and into the cooking water. That's why it's a good idea to use cooking water to thin purées — it returns some of the nutrients to the meal. You can also add them, diluted with fresh water, to a sippy cup and your baby can consume them between meals. To retain the maximum amount of nutrients, use fresh produce within a few days of purchase, cook fruits and vegetables with their skins on and prepare baby food as close to feeding time as possible.

Buy organic apples

2½ cups	water, approx. (see Tips, left)	625 mL
1½ cups	red lentils, rinsed	375 mL
1	Gala apple, cored and coarsely chopped	1

1. In a saucepan, combine water, lentils and apple. Bring to a boil over medium heat. Cover, reduce heat to low and simmer, stirring occasionally and adding more water if necessary to prevent sticking, until lentils are soft, about 25 minutes.

2. Transfer to a blender or use an immersion blender in the saucepan. Purée until smooth. Let cool until warm to the touch or transfer to an airtight container and refrigerate for up to 3 days or freeze for up to 1 month.

Nutrients per serving (¼ cup/50 mL)

Calories	35	Dietary fiber	2.2 g
Protein	2.3 g	Sodium	1.9 mg
Total fat	0.1 g	Calcium	6.6 mg
Saturated fat	0.0 g	Iron	0.8 mg
Carbohydrates	6.6 g	Vitamin C	0.9 mg

Not just for babies

For a remarkable textural contrast, combine this purée with its chunkier predecessor. Before puréeing, set aside 1 cup (250 mL) of the cooked lentils and apples, then purée the balance. In a saucepan, over low heat, combine the chunkier version with ½ cup (125 mL) of the purée. Stir in 1 tsp (5 mL) chopped fresh chives and 1 tbsp (15 mL) chopped tomatoes. Enjoy as a side dish at your next meal.

Celery Root and Chicken Purée

Your children will love the smooth, potato-like texture of celery root, not to mention its mild celery flavor.

Makes about 1¼ cups (300 mL)

Chef Jordan's Tips

Don't be scared of celery root. Also known as celeriac, it should be firm to the touch; if there's a little bit of give, it isn't fresh. Wash the celeriac thoroughly before peeling to avoid getting dirt on the flesh. In the absence of celery root, a combination of celery and parsnip does a fabulous job of mimicking its texture and flavor. Be sure to peel your celery to ensure a smooth texture in the final product.

Nutrition Tip

Celery root provides a good range of minerals, including phosphorus, which every cell of your baby's body requires to function normally. Eighty-five per cent of your baby's phosphorus is found in his bones and teeth.

1 cup	water	250 mL
½ cup	diced peeled celery root	125 mL
4 oz	boneless skinless chicken breast, cut in half	125 g

1. In a saucepan, combine water, celery root and chicken and bring to a boil over medium heat. Reduce heat to low and simmer until chicken is no longer pink inside and celery root is fork tender, about 20 minutes.

2. Transfer to a blender or use an immersion blender in the saucepan. Purée until smooth. Let cool until warm to the touch. Serve immediately or transfer to an airtight container and refrigerate for up to 3 days or freeze for up to 1 month.

Nutrients per serving (¼ cup/50 mL)	
Calories 52	Dietary fiber . . . . . . 0.5 g
Protein . . . . 8.1 g	Sodium . . . . 44.9 mg
Total fat . . . . 1.0 g	Calcium . . . . 15.9 mg
Saturated fat. . . . . . 0.3 g	Iron . . . . 0.4 mg
Carbohydrates. . . . . 2.3 g	Vitamin C. . . . . . . 2.0 mg

Not just for babies

Scoop some off to serve your baby and combine the remainder of this recipe with ½ cup (125 mL) whole milk or whipping (35%) cream to make a wonderful pasta sauce.

Sweet Peas, Lamb and Parsnip

The flavor of lamb can often overpower other ingredients. In this recipe, however, the sweetness of the parsnips and earthy tones of the peas work beautifully to tame the strong taste.

Makes about 1¼ cups (300 mL)

▪ ▪ ▪

Chef Jordan's Tips

When choosing a cut of lamb for a purée, it is important to choose a lean piece of meat. Don't use stewing meat in this recipe: It should only be used for stews or braising. Here, the meat doesn't cook long enough to break down the sinew.

Nutrition Tip

Lamb is a great protein source that contains significant amounts of iron. At about six months, infants have a greater need for both iron and protein to fuel the considerable growth that is happening at this stage in their development.

4 oz	boneless lamb loin, cubed (see Tips, left)	125 g
1 cup	water	250 mL
½ cup	frozen sweet peas	125 mL
¼ cup	coarsely chopped peeled parsnip	50 mL

1. In a saucepan, combine lamb, water, peas and parsnip. Bring to a boil over medium heat. Cover, reduce heat to low and simmer until parsnip is soft, about 10 minutes.

2. Transfer to a blender or use an immersion blender in the saucepan. Purée until smooth. Let cool until warm to the touch or transfer to an airtight container and refrigerate for up to 3 days or freeze for up to 1 month.

Nutrients per serving (¼ cup/50 mL)	
Calories 96	Dietary fiber . . . . . . 1.2 g
Protein . . . . 4.9 g	Sodium . . . . 48.6 mg
Total fat . . . . 6.7 g	Calcium . . . . 9.5 mg
Saturated fat. . . . . . 3.0 g	Iron . . . . 0.7 mg
Carbohydrates. . . . . 4.1 g	Vitamin C. . . . . . . 3.0 mg

Not just for babies

Sorry folks. This one really is just for babies. Freeze any extra to have on hand for future meals.

Chicken and Red Lentils

This Indian-inspired combination is a hit with babies, and Mom and Dad enjoy it, too.

Yield about 1½ cups (375 mL)

¾ cup	red lentils	175 mL
2 oz	boneless skinless chicken breast	60 g
1 cup	water	250 mL

1. In a sieve, rinse lentils under cold running water until water runs clear. Drain well.

2. In a saucepan, combine lentils, chicken and water. Bring to a boil over medium heat. Reduce heat to low and simmer, stirring occasionally, until chicken is no longer pink inside, lentils are soft and most of the water has been absorbed, about 25 minutes.

3. Transfer to a blender or use an immersion blender in the saucepan. Purée until smooth. Let cool until warm to the touch or transfer to an airtight container and refrigerate for up to 3 days or freeze for up to 1 month.

Chef Jordan's Tips

With my love of French cuisine it's not difficult to guess that my favorite lentil is the French Puy. Small and green-gray in color, this legume stands up against any hearty braise like an osso bucco or beef Bourguignon. Give it a try the next time you're shopping for a lentil, or substitute it for the red lentils in this recipe.

Nutrition Tip

Chicken, like all meats, contains all eight essential amino acids, including phenylalanine and methionine. Phenylalanine is specifically responsible for the positive brain chemicals that keep your baby's alertness levels and potential for learning at its height. Methionine's sulfur content opens detoxification pathways that help baby's body eliminate heavy metals.

Nutrients per serving (¼ cup/50 mL)	
Calories 92	Dietary fiber . . . . . . 1.3 g
Protein . . . . 8.4 g	Sodium . . . . 51.7 mg
Total fat . . . . 0.2 g	Calcium . . . . 11.2 mg
Saturated fat. . . . . . 0.0 g	Iron . . . . 0.8 mg
Carbohydrates. . . . 13.6 g	Vitamin C. . . . . . . 0.0 mg

Not just for babies

As Jonah gets older, Tamar and I are able to expand the variety of foods he eats without him realizing it. Often I'll make "chicken wraps" for him filled with chicken lentil purée, grilled chicken, tomatoes and cheese and seared like a grilled cheese sandwich. We enjoy them together!

Grilled Chicken and Avocado

"Ladies and gentleman, we have a winner!" I love the flavor combination of chicken and avocado and usually enjoy it at least once a week.

Makes about 2 cups (500 mL)

∎ ∎ ∎

Chef Jordan's Tips

If timing is an issue, a store-bought rotisserie chicken would be a good substitute for grilled chicken in this recipe. Remove skin and all bones and pieces of cartilage before chopping. When buying a cooked chicken, choose one that hasn't been sitting under the heat lamp too long as it tends to be quite dry.

Nutrition Tip

Although your baby needs a diet that is higher in fat in infancy, he does not need an overabundance of saturated fat. Removing the skin from chicken is a practice that will serve him well throughout life. Even though dark meat has a little more fat than white, it also contains more minerals, so feel free to substitute dark meat for the breast in this recipe.

• **Preheat barbecue to high or 500°F (260°C)**

8 oz	boneless skinless chicken breast	250 g
1¼ cups	coarsely chopped pitted peeled avocado (about 1)	300 mL
½ cup	water	125 mL

1. On a preheated barbecue, grill chicken breast until well browned, about 10 minutes. Turn and cook until no longer pink inside, 3 to 4 minutes. Let cool until warm to the touch, about 15 minutes. Cut into cubes.

2. In a saucepan, combine chicken, avocado and water. Bring to a boil over medium heat. Transfer to a blender or use an immersion blender in the saucepan. Purée until smooth. Let cool until warm to the touch. Serve immediately or transfer to an airtight container and refrigerate for up to 3 days or freeze for up to 1 month.

Nutrients per serving (¼ cup/50 mL)	
Calories 89	Dietary fiber . . . . . . 1.6 g
Protein . . . . 10.2 g	Sodium . . . . 25.2 mg
Total fat . . . . 4.6 g	Calcium . . . . 8.0 mg
Saturated fat. . . . . . 0.8 g	Iron . . . . 0.5 mg
Carbohydrates. . . . . 2.0 g	Vitamin C. . . . . . . 2.3 mg

Not just for babies

The addition of chopped tomatoes and Cheddar cheese transforms this purée into an awesome burrito stuffing. Simply roll in a flour tortilla and bake at 300°F (150°C) until cheese is melted, about 5 minutes.

White Navy Bean and Beef Tenderloin Purée

The flavors of white beans and beef belong together — that's why the combination is a classic.

Makes about 2¼ cups (550 mL)

■ ■ ■

Chef Jordan's Tips
Use any dried white bean, such as navy, Great Northern or cannellini, in this recipe.

Nutrition Tip
This purée provides zinc from both the beans and the beef. Zinc is involved in more body functions than any other mineral. Adequate levels of zinc are necessary for proper immune function and to decrease the risk of infections. It is also essential to help your body heal cuts and scrapes.

3 cups	water	750 mL
½ cup	dried white navy beans, soaked, drained and rinsed (see page 77)	125 mL
¾ cup	coarsely chopped peeled carrot	175 mL
4 oz	beef tenderloin	125 g

1. In a saucepan, combine water, beans, carrot and beef. Bring to a boil over medium heat. Reduce heat to low and simmer until beans are fork tender, about 75 minutes.

2. Transfer to a blender or use an immersion blender in the saucepan. Purée until smooth. Let cool until warm to the touch or transfer to an airtight container and refrigerate for up to 3 days or freeze for up to 1 month.

Nutrients per serving (¼ cup/50 mL)	
Calories 40	Dietary fiber . . . . . . 1.3 g
Protein . . . . 4.1 g	Sodium . . . . 18.0 g
Total fat . . . . 1.1 g	Calcium . . . . 17.2 g
Saturated fat. . . . . . 0.3 g	Iron . . . . 0.5 mg
Carbohydrates. . . . . 3.6 g	Vitamin C. . . . . . . 0.6 mg

Not just for babies
Before puréeing, set aside ½ cup (125 mL) of the beans, leaving the beef for the baby. Combine with 2 cups (500 mL) arugula and toss in a horseradish vinaigrette. The salad is awesome.

Cook Your Own Beans

Storing

Once cooked, beans (and chickpeas) should be covered and stored in the refrigerator, where they will keep for up to 4 days. Cooked beans can be frozen in an airtight container for up to 6 months.

When a recipe calls for cooked beans, such as navy, cannellini or chickpeas, you have two options: You can cook dried beans from scratch or use canned beans, which produce a similar result. However, canned beans usually contain significant amounts of sodium. If you are using canned beans in any of our recipes, be sure to rinse them thoroughly under cold running water to remove as much of the added salt as possible, or purchase a brand with no salt added (for more on canned beans, see page 105).

While it is not difficult to prepare dried beans from scratch, you do need to plan ahead because they need to be soaked before they are cooked. The following instructions can be adjusted to suit the quantity of beans (or chickpeas) you wish to cook — it can be halved, doubled or tripled. A good rule of thumb is that 1 cup (250 mL) dried beans makes 2 cups (500 mL) cooked. Although the sizes of canned beans vary, standard cans usually range in size from 14 oz (398 mL) to 19 oz (540 mL), each providing about 2 cups (500 mL) of cooked beans. A little more or less usually doesn't matter in a recipe.

Long soak: In a bowl, combine 1 cup (250 mL) dried beans (or chickpeas) and 3 cups (750 mL) water. Set aside for at least 6 hours or overnight. Drain and rinse thoroughly with cold water. Beans are now ready for cooking.

Quick soak: In a saucepan, combine beans (or chickpeas) and water. Cover and bring to a boil. Boil for 3 minutes. Turn off heat and soak for 1 hour. Drain and rinse thoroughly under cold water. Beans are now ready to cook.

To cook soaked beans (or chickpeas): In a saucepan, combine 1 cup (250 mL) soaked beans and 3 cups (750 mL) fresh cold water. Bring to a boil over medium-high heat. Reduce heat to low and simmer until beans are tender, 45 minutes to 1 hour, depending upon the variety.

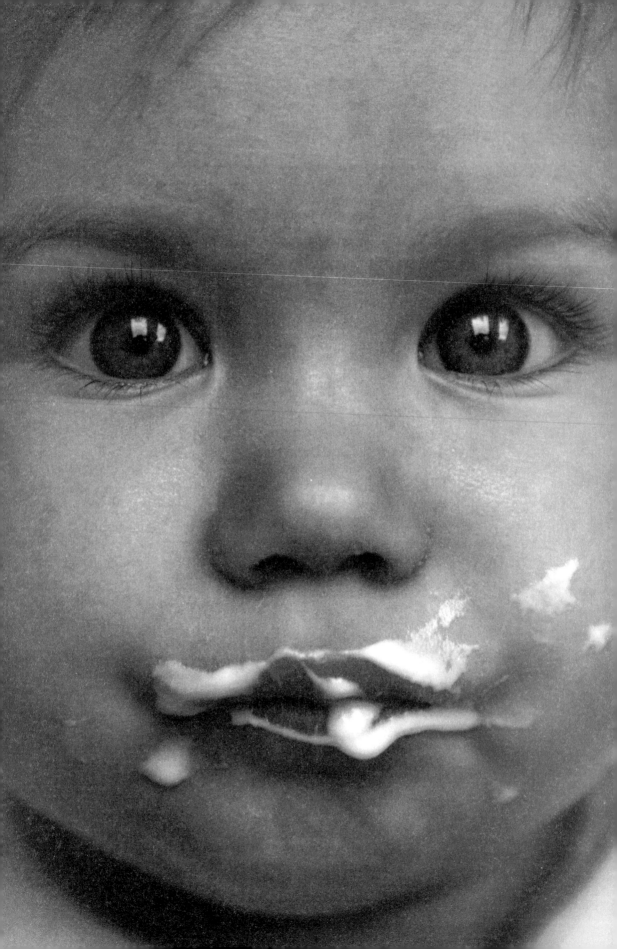

Establishing Preferences
(9 to 12 Months)

Introduction 80

Dishes with Dairy
Vanilla Bean Yogurt 82
Stewed Leeks with Butter 83
The Best Eggplant Parmesan 84
Brussels Sprout Gratin 85
Mediterranean Fried Eggplant 86
Diced Potato Gratin 87
Poached Garlic Cloves with
   Fresh Thyme and Sour Cream 88

Grains and Fruit
Summer Cherry and Quinoa 89
Millet Cereal with Crushed
   Bananas and Sour Cream 90

Vegetable Combos
Egg and Sweet Pepper Fried Rice . . . 91
Bok Choy with Fresh Ginger 92
Brussels Sprouts with Bacon 93
Oven-Roasted Cherry Tomato
   Purée 94

Turnip and Parsnip "Smash" 95
Red Cabbage, Fennel and
   Apple Purée 96
Roasted Onion Soubise 97
Potato, Parsnip and Chicken Soup
   with Chive Parsley "Pistou" 98
Chive Parsley "Pistou" 99
Ratatouille Vegetables 101
Sautéed Chard with Apples 102

Legumes
Fresh Soy Bean Hummus 103
White Bean and Fennel Purée 104

Meat Combos
Oven-Roasted Chicken with
   Dried Apricots 106
Chicken with Roasted
   Butternut Squash and Leeks 108
Pork Tenderloin and Peaches 109
Beef Tenderloin and Dates 110
Lamb with Parsnips and
   Dried Cranberries 111

Introduction

Throughout the nine- to twelve-month period, your child's intake of breast milk or formula will decline and solid foods will replace this source of calories. Once your baby reaches eight or nine months, she may be more assertive at displaying her individuality, especially at mealtime. She is likely to be more definite about the food she likes and at times may even refuse to eat a particular food. It is common for babies of this age to tightly purse their lips, turn their heads away so the food you are offering ends up in their ear, and even throw food. This behavior can be very frustrating to parents who just want to make sure their baby gets fed.

Allowing your baby to exert some independence can go a long way toward keeping the peace at mealtime. Give your baby a small, rounded spoon to experiment with, and place some mashed food directly on her tray so she can try feeding herself. Again, every baby progresses at her own rate, so take your cues from her when determining the next step. It is your job as a parent to provide appropriate nourishing foods at each stage of your baby's life, but it is your baby who decides how much of these foods she will eat at a sitting. By respecting your baby's unspoken messages about hunger and fullness, you are helping her to establish a lifelong pattern of healthy eating.

At this age, your baby will enjoy eating slightly lumpier foods. If you make the transition to more textured food gradually, you'll provide her with time to adjust. Continue to use all the recipes from Chapter 1, but instead of puréeing, try pulsing the food to produce a coarser texture. You can even mash it with a fork or cut it into a fine mince, depending on your baby's preferences. In this chapter, we have included recipes that use egg yolks, cheese and yogurt, which are appropriate for this age group. Adding these new foods to your baby's diet will help you to continue expanding your baby's palate, as well as her nutritional intake.

This age is also the time to introduce finger foods, as your baby's dexterity is increasing. Good options here include pieces of well-cooked (then cooled) vegetables such as turnip, squash and carrots and soft fruits such as peaches, pears and bananas. Make sure the pieces are soft enough to be mashed against the roof of your baby's mouth and small enough to prevent choking. Finger foods cut into $\frac{1}{4}$-inch (0.5 cm) square pieces (dice) should be small enough for her to scoop up with her fingers, but even so, you'll need to constantly supervise when your baby is eating to make sure she doesn't choke on anything. Continuing to offer her a wide variety of foods with different colors, tastes and textures will help her to accept new flavors and the new foods to come.

Your baby may show some interest in drinking from your glass and may like to try her own sippy cup. Fresh water is the best thing to put in her cup. Juice, even that made from pure fruits, is still a highly concentrated sugar. It isn't necessary for a child whose diet includes puréed or mashed whole fruit. Even though she may not get too much out of the sippy cup at this point, juice may decrease her appetite for the nutrient-dense solid foods you have prepared. Now and throughout their toddler years, encourage your child to eat whole foods and drink fresh water for optimal health.

Vanilla Bean Yogurt

When it comes to vanilla, nothing beats the bean. Pure vanilla extract makes an acceptable substitute (see Tips, below) but the flavor of imitations pales in comparison. Your baby will love this, not only plain and simple but also added to fruit purées or hot cereals.

Makes about 2 cups (500 mL)

■ ■ ■

| 1 | vanilla bean or 1 tsp (5 mL) pure vanilla extract (see Tips, left) | 1 |
| 2 cups | plain full-fat yogurt | 500 mL |

1. Using a paring knife, cut vanilla bean in half lengthwise, releasing the seeds. Scrape seeds into a bowl. Add yogurt and mix well. Serve immediately or transfer to an airtight container and refrigerate for up to 3 days.

Chef Jordan's Tips

Reserve the pods to flavor sugar or salt.

Vanilla beans can be purchased in well-stocked supermarkets and specialty shops. If unavailable, pure vanilla extract, with no alcohol, will substitute well. Please avoid using artificial extracts and opt instead for pure extract, which although more expensive, tastes so much better.

Nutrition Tip

Be sure to look for whole yogurt that contains the friendly bacteria *Lactobacillus acidophilus*, which is found in large amounts in your baby's intestines. These probiotics are fierce protectors of your baby's immunity and should be replaced constantly, especially if your baby has recently been prescribed antibiotics.

Nutrients per serving (1/4 cup/50 mL)

Calories 39	Dietary fiber . . . . . . 0.0 g
Protein . . . . 2.1 g	Sodium . . . . 28.2 mg
Total fat . . . . 2.0 g	Calcium . . . . 74.2 mg
Saturated fat. . . . . . 1.3 g	Iron . . . . 0.0 mg
Carbohydrates. . . . . 2.9 g	Vitamin C. . . . . . . 0.3 mg

Not just for babies

This yogurt makes a wonderful canvas for an appetizer. How about chicken skewers with a drizzle of Vanilla Bean Yogurt? If you ask in advance, your butcher will usually assemble skewers for you. Ask him or her to place the chicken on one end of the wooden skewer. Leaving the other end bare will make it easy to pass them around as appetizers.

Stewed Leeks with Butter

If you and your family have never tried leeks, try this simple recipe. Leeks have a very mild flavor, unlike their pungent relatives, onions. Their pleasing delicate flavor is impossible to duplicate!

Makes about 1 cup (250 mL)

■ ■ ■

Chef Jordan's Tips

Leeks can be sandy but are easy to clean. Cut them lengthwise, rinse thoroughly under cold running water and pat dry.

I'm fortunate to live in a region where, in the spring, I can find wild leeks, also known as ramps. Ramps have a delicate onion flavor with a slight hint of garlic, and an equal quantity would work beautifully in this recipe.

Nutrition Tip

A member of the allium family, leeks are the cousins of onions and garlic. This family of vegetables contains sulfur compounds that appear to have a very positive effect on your health. Among other benefits, these compounds support the normal function of the liver, helping it to detoxify your baby's body from possible contaminants.

1 tbsp	unsalted butter	15 mL
2¼ cups	chopped leeks, white part only (see Tips, left)	550 mL

1. In a saucepan, melt butter over low heat. Add leeks, cover and cook, stirring often, until very soft, about 30 minutes.

2. Transfer to a blender or use an immersion blender in the saucepan. Purée to your baby's preferred consistency, pulsing for a chunkier consistency. Let cool until warm to the touch or transfer to an airtight container and refrigerate for up to 3 days.

Nutrients per serving (¼ cup/50 mL)	
Calories 52	Dietary fiber . . . . . . 0.9 g
Protein . . . . 1.8 g	Sodium . . . . 0.4 mg
Total fat . . . . 2.9 g	Calcium . . . . 36.2 mg
Saturated fat. . . . . 1.8 g	Iron . . . . 2.4 mg
Carbohydrates. . . . . 5.3 g	Vitamin C. . . . . . 23.8 mg

Not just for babies

The next time you're making pizza at home, try these stewed leeks as a topping. Just spread on top after you take the pizza out of the oven.

The Best Eggplant Parmesan

This versatile purée, embellished with roasted tomatoes and basil, is a hit with babies, but Mom and Dad will love it, too!

Makes about 3 cups (750 mL)

■ ■ ■

Chef Jordan's Tips
From time to time, I'll come across an eggplant that is a little bitter and that needs to be "sweated." Slice the eggplant, sprinkle with kosher salt and let it stand in a colander for an hour or so, which draws out quite a bit of liquid. After a thorough rinsing under cold running water, pat the eggplant dry with a paper towel.

Nutrition Tip
Eggplant purée has a gelatinous and velvety mouth feel. Introducing food that has an unusual texture, like eggplant, to your baby at this point may increase the chances that he will accept new and more exotic foods as he grows older. Expanding your baby's palette now will predispose him to enjoy a wide variety of foods as an adult, providing the nutritional benefit that comes from a varied diet.

- Preheat oven to 350°F (180°C)
- Ovenproof skillet

2 tbsp	extra virgin olive oil (approx)	25 mL
8 cups	coarsely chopped eggplant (about 1 medium, 2 lbs/1 kg)	2 L
1½ cups	Oven-Roasted Cherry Tomato Purée (see recipe, page 94)	375 mL
⅓ cup	freshly grated Parmesan cheese	75 mL
2	basil leaves	2

1. In ovenproof skillet, heat oil over medium-high heat. Add eggplant, in batches, and cook, stirring, until golden brown, adding more oil as necessary, about 5 minutes per batch. Return eggplant to the skillet. Stir in tomato purée and cheese. Bake in preheated oven until eggplant is very soft and sauce is boiling, about 35 minutes.

2. Add basil leaves. Transfer to a blender or to a bowl and use an immersion blender. Purée to your baby's preferred consistency, pulsing for a chunkier consistency. Let cool until warm to the touch or transfer to an airtight container and refrigerate for up to 3 days.

Nutrients per serving (¼ cup/50 mL)	
Calories 60	Dietary fiber . . . . . . 3.1 g
Protein . . . . 2.0 g	Sodium . . . . 35.9 mg
Total fat . . . . 3.6 g	Calcium . . . . 35.2 mg
Saturated fat. . . . . 0.8 g	Iron . . . . 0.3 mg
Carbohydrates. . . . . 6.1 g	Vitamin C. . . . . . . 7.2 mg

Brussels Sprout Gratin

You won't believe these are the same Brussels sprouts your mom used to serve! Adding Parmesan cheese creates a match made in heaven.

Makes about 1 cup (250 mL)

∎ ∎ ∎

Chef Jordan's Tips

Typically found in late fall and winter, these tiny members of the cabbage family should be bright green and firm to the touch.

Nutrition Tip

Brussels sprouts are a cruciferous vegetable and part of the brassica family, which also includes its big brothers cabbage, broccoli and cauliflower. These vegetables are known for their cancer-fighting ability. Sulforaphane, a phytonutrient found in Brussels sprouts, enhances the activity of your baby's natural defense systems, protecting against many diseases.

- Preheat oven to 350°F (180°C)
- Casserole dish with lid

2 cups	coarsely chopped Brussels sprouts (about 6 oz/175 g)	500 mL
1/3 cup	freshly grated Parmesan cheese	75 mL
1/4 cup	water	50 mL
2 tbsp	sour cream	25 mL

1. In casserole dish, combine sprouts, cheese, water and sour cream. Stir well, cover and bake in preheated oven until sprouts are soft, about 1 hour.

2. Transfer to a blender or use an immersion blender in the dish. Purée to your baby's preferred consistency, pulsing for a chunkier consistency. Let cool until warm to the touch or transfer to an airtight container and refrigerate for up to 3 days.

Nutrients per serving (1/4 cup/50 mL)	
Calories 61	Dietary fiber . . . . . . 1.6 g
Protein . . . . 3.7 g	Sodium . . . . . . 112.5 mg
Total fat . . . . 3.1 g	Calcium . . . . 85.3 mg
Saturated fat. . . . . . 1.8 g	Iron . . . . 0.1 mg
Carbohydrates. . . . . 3.6 g	Vitamin C. . . . . . 37.5 mg

Not just for babies

Brussels Sprout Gratin is a great ingredient in turkey stuffing. Triple the recipe and add 2 cups (500 mL) diced bread, 3/4 cup (175 mL) chopped fresh herbs, 1/2 cup (125 mL) chopped celery, 1/2 cup (125 mL) chopped carrots, 1/2 cup (125 mL) diced sweet onion and 1 tsp (5 mL) each salt and freshly ground black pepper.

Mediterranean Fried Eggplant

While living in Israel, I would frequently visit Tamar's cousins who had twin daughters. They often served this purée to their babies and they loved it. I'm sure your baby will love it, too.

**Makes about
2 cups (500 mL)**

■ ■ ■

Chef Jordan's Tips

Cooking in batches helps maintain pan temperature. Overloading tends to lower the temperature, which in this case can result in eggplant with a soggy texture.

Substitute other fresh herbs such as oregano, parsley, chervil, tarragon or dill for the basil.

Nutrition Tip

When selecting eggplant, choose those that are heavy for their size and have smooth, shiny skins free of scars and bruising, which can indicate that the flesh inside is damaged. Keep the eggplant whole until you are ready to use it because it deteriorates quickly when cut. A fresh eggplant will last for up to one week in the crisper of the refrigerator or for just a few days at room temperature.

● Preheat oven to 350°F (180°C)

½ cup	extra virgin olive oil, divided	125 mL
2 lbs	eggplant, cut into 1-inch (2.5 cm) thick round slices (about 1 medium)	1 kg
⅓ cup	freshly grated Parmesan cheese	75 mL
2 tbsp	thinly sliced basil leaves	25 mL

1. In a large skillet, heat 2 tbsp (25 mL) of the oil over medium-high heat. Add eggplant in batches and cook (see Tips, left), turning once, until golden brown on both sides, about 4 minutes per side. Transfer to a plate lined with paper towel. Add more oil and reheat pan between batches as necessary.

2. Add Parmesan and basil. Transfer to a blender or to a bowl or cup and use an immersion blender. Purée to your baby's preferred consistency, pulsing for a chunkier consistency. Let cool until warm to the touch or transfer to an airtight container and refrigerate for up to 3 days.

Nutrients per serving (¼ cup/50 mL)	
Calories 174	Dietary fiber . . . . . . 3.9 g
Protein . . . . 2.4 g	Sodium . . . . 50.8 mg
Total fat . . . . 15.9 g	Calcium . . . . 46.4 mg
Saturated fat. . . . . . 2.7 g	Iron . . . . 0.3 mg
Carbohydrates. . . . . 6.6 g	Vitamin C. . . . . . . 2.6 mg

Not just for babies

There isn't a Mediterranean meal I prepare for my family that doesn't include this dish. Adults enjoy it just as much as babies.

Diced Potato Gratin

I'll never forget the time the legendary chef Paul Bocuse came to Pascal in Newport Beach, Calif., the restaurant where I was chef. He taught me this very simple potato recipe. It is so easy to make and encapsulates the essence of French cuisine: simple ingredients, made with lots of love. Your baby will love it, and the recipe makes enough for the rest of the family to enjoy as well.

Makes about 4 cups (1 L)

Chef Jordan's Tips

Cooks are taught to store cut potatoes in water to avoid oxidization, but it also draws out the starch. In this case starch is good because it helps the milk to thicken. So when making this recipe, dice potatoes and use them immediately.

Try Yukon Gold or fingerling potatoes.

Nutrition Tip

The beneficial nutrients in potatoes are found in both the flesh and the skin. These nutrients include flavonoids, which may help to protect your baby from respiratory problems such as asthma, and a recently discovered compound called kukoamine, which appears to keep blood pressure in check.

* Potato Masher

2¹/₂ cups	whole milk	625 mL
1 tbsp	unsalted butter	15 mL
2 cups	finely diced baking potatoes, unpeeled (see Tips, left)	500 mL
²/₃ cup	freshly grated Parmesan cheese	150 mL

1. In a saucepan, combine milk and butter. Bring to a simmer over medium heat. Stir in potatoes. Reduce heat to low and simmer until potatoes are fork tender, about 20 minutes.

2. Stir in Parmesan. Using a potato masher, mash to your baby's preferred consistency. Let cool until warm to the touch or transfer to an airtight container and refrigerate for up to 3 days.

Nutrients per serving (¹/₄ cup/50 mL)	
Calories 66	Dietary fiber . . . . . . 0.6 g
Protein . . . . 3.1 g	Sodium . . . . 66.4 mg
Total fat . . . . 3.0 g	Calcium . . . . 84.3 mg
Saturated fat. . . . . . 1.8 g	Iron . . . . 0.3 mg
Carbohydrates. . . . . 6.9 g	Vitamin C. . . . . . . 5.6 mg

Not just for babies
Make this dish in a large quantity because everyone will enjoy it as much as Baby. Serve to Mom and Dad without mashing.

Poached Garlic Cloves with Fresh Thyme and Sour Cream

I understand you may be reluctant to serve your baby a purée of garlic. However, when garlic is poached with aromatics, such as fresh thyme, it becomes sweet and quite mild. When combined with sour cream, the texture and flavor is similar to mashed potatoes.

Makes about ¾ cup (175 mL)

■ ■ ■

Chef Jordan's Tips

Garlic skins come off easily after the cloves are poached whole. Bring water to a boil and blanch the garlic cloves for 3 to 5 minutes. The skins will easily come off and the garlic will remain raw.

Nutrition Tip

One of garlic's most studied properties is that of infection fighter, due to its allicin content. Quite a few studies have shown that allicin acts as a broad-spectrum antibacterial that can battle a wide range of pathogens, such as *E. coli* and salmonella, which can be brought into the home environment on food products. Always consult your doctor if you think your baby is sick, but add some garlic to her diet, too, for good measure.

1¼ cups	cloves garlic, unpeeled (see Tips, left)	300 mL
1 cup	water	250 mL
1	sprig thyme	1
2 tbsp	full-fat sour cream	25 mL

1. In a saucepan, combine garlic, water and thyme. Bring to a boil over medium heat. Reduce heat to low and simmer until garlic is fork tender, about 15 minutes. Set aside until cool enough to handle.

2. Squeeze each clove of garlic to remove skin and round "stem" at one end of clove (both should remove quite easily) and place in a bowl. Add sour cream and mash to desired consistency. Serve immediately or transfer to an airtight container and refrigerate for up to 3 days or freeze for up to 1 month.

Nutrients per serving (¼ cup/50 mL)	
Calories 105	Dietary fiber . . . . . . 1.2 g
Protein . . . . 4.0 g	Sodium . . . . 15.4 mg
Total fat . . . . 2.0 g	Calcium . . . . . . 112.7 mg
Saturated fat. . . . . . 1.2 g	Iron . . . . 1.0 mg
Carbohydrates. . . . 19.1 g	Vitamin C. . . . . . 18.1 mg

Not just for babies

I often use this recipe as a garnish for steaks.

Summer Cherry and Quinoa

I wish there was a secret to pitting cherries, but there isn't! It's messy and time consuming but well worth the fuss! The fresh cherries complement the quinoa beautifully in this recipe.

Makes about 1½ cups (375 mL)

■ ■ ■

Chef Jordan's Tips

Bing cherries, which are available in spring and throughout summer, are my favorite cherry. This dark purple, firm fruit has unique contrasting flavors of sweet and sour.

With a slight nutty flavor, quinoa can easily substitute for couscous or rice in most recipes.

Nutrition Tip

Cherries contain flavonoids, compounds that are very high in antioxidant activity. Among their many benefits, flavonoids appear to have anti-inflammatory properties and may help your baby to fight an allergic response.

Buy organic cherries

1 cup	pitted Bing or other sweet cherries	250 mL
1 cup	water	250 mL
¾ cup	cooked quinoa (see recipe, page 48)	175 mL

1. In a saucepan, combine cherries and water. Bring to a boil over medium heat and cook, stirring often, until almost falling apart, about 5 minutes.

2. Transfer to a blender or use an immersion blender in the saucepan. Purée until smooth. Return to the saucepan, if necessary, and add quinoa. Place over low heat and simmer, stirring occasionally, until thick, about 20 minutes. Let cool until warm to the touch or transfer to an airtight container and refrigerate for up to 3 days.

Nutrients per serving (¼ cup/50 mL)	
Calories 20	Dietary fiber . . . . . . 0.6 g
Protein . . . . 0.4 g	Sodium . . . . 1.7 mg
Total fat . . . . 0.3 g	Calcium . . . . 5.6 mg
Saturated fat . . . . . . 0.0 g	Iron . . . . 0.1 mg
Carbohydrates . . . . . 4.8 g	Vitamin C . . . . 0.8 mg

Not just for babies

It always amazes me how so many of my baby food concoctions become an instant adult classic. For instance, one of my favorite breakfasts is muesli, brightened by the addition of Summer Cherry and Quinoa. I love the flavor and color the cherries impart to the milk, which I love to drink when all the cereal is gone. You can also try this with cottage cheese and yogurt.

Millet Cereal with Crushed Bananas and Sour Cream

This is a cereal for both baby and family. The Wagman family often substitutes millet cereal for porridge in the morning.

Makes about 3¼ cups (800 mL)

■ ■ ■

Chef Jordan's Tips

Sour cream adds a unique citrus undertone to this cereal. Alternatively, an equal quantity of creamy goat cheese would have a similar effect.

Nutrition Tip

Millet is a wonderful grain for your baby. It is gluten-free and hypoallergenic and has a nice mild flavor. It is also very digestible. Millet contains the mineral manganese, which is involved in many enzyme systems in the body, including the antioxidant enzyme superoxide dismutase. This extremely important enzyme helps prevent free radicals from destroying cells and protects the body from damage and inflammation.

3½ cups	water	875 mL
¾ cup	millet flour (see page 51)	175 mL
1 cup	coarsely chopped bananas (about 2)	250 mL
2 tbsp	full-fat sour cream	25 mL
1 tsp	alcohol-free pure vanilla extract	5 mL

1. In a saucepan, bring water to a boil over medium heat. Slowly add millet flour, whisking constantly to avoid lumps. Add bananas and cook, whisking, until thick (almost porridge-like), about 10 minutes. Remove from heat and set aside, covered, until very thick, about 20 minutes.

2. Stir in sour cream and vanilla until thoroughly combined. Serve immediately or transfer to an airtight container and refrigerate for up to 3 days. To serve, reheat ½ cup (125 mL) of cooked cereal with ¼ cup (50 mL) water in a saucepan over low heat just until warm.

Nutrients per serving (¼ cup/50 mL)	
Calories 21	Dietary fiber . . . . . . 0.5 g
Protein . . . . 0.3 g	Sodium . . . . 2.9 mg
Total fat . . . . 0.5 g	Calcium . . . . 4.4 mg
Saturated fat. . . . . . 0.3 g	Iron . . . . 0.1 mg
Carbohydrates. . . . . 4.1 g	Vitamin C. . . . . . . 1.5 mg

Not just for babies

For Mom and Dad, a light drizzle of maple syrup or sprinkling of brown sugar makes a sweet, nutritious breakfast. Enjoy!

Egg and Sweet Pepper Fried Rice

This is a great way to introduce your baby to the wonders of Chinese food.

**Makes about
2½ cups (625 mL)**

■ ■ ■

Chef Jordan's Tips
Fried rice is really a
blank canvas, an
opportunity to be
creative with produce
you have around that
might need to be eaten,
also known in my
family as "the fridge
clean meal." From
cabbage to spinach and
sweet potato to corn,
I've made fried rice
using just about
anything. Experiment;
you may come up with
something excellent.

Nutrition Tip
Ounce for ounce, red
peppers have even more
vitamin C than oranges.
Vitamin C is an
antioxidant that
neutralizes free radicals,
which can damage
developing artery walls.
It keeps the arteries
smooth and helps
prevent the buildup of
plaque and cholesterol.

2 tbsp	extra virgin olive oil, divided	25 mL
½ cup	finely diced red bell pepper	125 mL
½ cup	finely diced sweet onion	125 mL
1 tsp	minced gingerroot	5 mL
¾ cup	basmati rice, rinsed	175 mL
1¼ cups	water	300 mL
2	egg yolks, whisked	2

1. In a saucepan, heat half of the oil over medium heat.
   Add pepper, onion and ginger, and sauté until onion
   is translucent. Stir in rice. Add water and bring to a
   rapid boil. Cover, reduce heat to low and simmer for
   5 minutes. Remove from heat and set aside, covered,
   until liquid is absorbed, about 25 minutes.

2. In a large skillet, heat remaining oil over high heat.
   Add egg yolks, swirl and cook until they form a thin
   "omelet." Stir in rice mixture. Cook, without
   stirring, for 3 minutes. Stir well and cook until
   mixture is warm throughout, about 5 minutes.
   Purée to your baby's preferred consistency, pulsing
   for a chunkier consistency. Let cool until warm to
   the touch or transfer to an airtight container and
   refrigerate for up to 2 days.

Nutrients per serving (¼ cup/50 mL)			
Calories	66	Dietary fiber	0.4 g
Protein	1.2 g	Sodium	3.2 mg
Total fat	3.7 g	Calcium	7.7 mg
Saturated fat	0.7 g	Iron	0.2 mg
Carbohydrates	6.8 g	Vitamin C	10.7 mg

Not just for babies
Serve this as a side dish for Mom and Dad.

Bok Choy with Fresh Ginger

Bok choy and ginger is a classic Chinese flavor combination.

**Makes about
1¾ cups (425 mL)**

■ ■ ■

Chef Jordan's Tips
One of my favorite
vegetables is gai-lan, or
Chinese broccoli. With
a very thin, tender stalk
(much more tender than
traditional broccoli) and
luscious green leaves,
it's a vegetable your
kids will easily take to.
Give it a try in place
of the bok choy. It's
a winner here!

Nutrition Tip
Trains, planes and
automobiles! Ginger has
the amazing property of
calming motion sickness
and nausea in sensitive
tummies. When you
travel, pack this
soothing purée to lessen
these unpleasant effects.

¼ cup	water	50 mL
1 lb	bok choy, chopped (about 4 cups/1 L)	500 g
2 tsp	minced gingerroot	10 mL

1. In a saucepan, bring water to a boil over high heat. Stir in bok choy and gingerroot. Cover, reduce heat to low and cook until soft, about 20 minutes.
2. Transfer to a blender or use an immersion blender in the saucepan. Purée to your baby's preferred consistency, pulsing for a chunkier consistency. Let cool until warm to the touch or transfer to an airtight container and refrigerate for up to 3 days.

Nutrients per serving (¼ cup/50 mL)

Calories	10	Dietary fiber	0.7 g
Protein	1.1 g	Sodium	46.7 mg
Total fat	0.2 g	Calcium	75.3 mg
Saturated fat	0.0 g	Iron	0.6 mg
Carbohydrates	1.7 g	Vitamin C	32.2 mg

Not just for babies
Before puréeing, remove some bok choy for
Mom and Dad and add 1 tbsp (15 mL) soy sauce
and a dash of rice vinegar for added flavor. This
is excellent over cooked brown rice. When it
comes to soy sauce, my preference is tamari.
Tamari is typically made from soy beans, as
opposed to many Chinese and Japanese soy
sauces, which are frequently made with various
other grains, including wheat.

Brussels Sprouts with Bacon

Just because you didn't like these mini-cabbages when you were growing up doesn't mean they won't be one of your baby's favorites. Your parents just didn't know how to make them taste great! A little bit of bacon makes a big difference.

**Makes about
1 cup (250 mL)**

■ ■ ■

Chef Jordan's Tips
Nitrates, which are found in most processed meats, are added as a preservative. Concerns have been raised about their long-term safety because it appears they may have carcinogenic effects. That's why I recommend using bacon that is nitrate-free.

Nutrition Tip
In order to reduce the dangers associated with nitrates in processed and deli meats, some manufacturers who add nitrates to bacon are also adding vitamin C to their product. Consumption of vitamin C has been shown to lessen the negative effects of these potentially cancer-causing chemicals. However, the safest strategy is to make it a rule to use organic, nitrate-free meats.

1 oz	nitrate-free bacon, minced (about 1 slice)	30 g
2 cups	coarsely chopped Brussels sprouts (about 6 oz/175 g)	500 mL
¼ cup	water	50 mL

1. In a saucepan, over medium heat, sauté bacon until crispy and brown, about 3 minutes. Stir in Brussels sprouts. Reduce heat to low and cook, stirring frequently to avoid browning, until soft, about 10 minutes. Add water and simmer until water has evaporated, about 5 minutes.

2. Transfer to a blender or use an immersion blender in the saucepan. Purée to your baby's preferred consistency, pulsing for a chunkier consistency. Let cool until warm to the touch or transfer to an airtight container and refrigerate for up to 3 days.

Nutrients per serving (¼ cup/50 mL)	
Calories 58	Dietary fiber . . . . . . 1.6 g
Protein . . . . 3.4 g	Sodium . . . . . . 168.4 mg
Total fat . . . . 3.4 g	Calcium . . . . 12.0 mg
Saturated fat. . . . . . 1.1 g	Iron . . . . 0.1 mg
Carbohydrates. . . . . 3.2 g	Vitamin C. . . . . . 37.5 mg

Not just for babies
After sautéing the Brussels sprouts, spoon off a serving for your baby, add a pinch of salt and pepper and serve warm. Purée the remainder for your baby to enjoy. This makes an excellent side dish with pork or beef.

Oven-Roasted Cherry Tomato Purée

You'll want to make this your new staple tomato sauce and get ride of store-bought imposters. For Baby, add to barley or rice to create an excellent meal.

Makes about 1½ cups (375 mL)

■ ■ ■

Chef Jordan's Tips

This recipe has a unique flavor specific to cherry, currant or grape tomatoes, but it also works with plum tomatoes. Cut plum tomatoes in half and roast until wilted but still retaining moisture, about 1 hour, then complete Step 2. Another great method of preparation is to grill whole plum tomatoes. Drizzle with a little olive oil and grill until nicely charred on all sides.

Nutrition Tip

Tomatoes are an excellent source of lycopene, a phytonutrient that is thought to have anti-cancer properties. Cooking heightens lycopene absorption, as does the addition of olive oil. The combination of fat and heat maximizes the free-radical-hunting ability of this nutrient.

- Preheat oven to 350°F (180°C)
- Ovenproof saucepan

1 lb	cherry tomatoes (about 2 cups/500 mL)	500 g
1 tsp	extra virgin olive oil	5 mL
2	sprigs fresh thyme	2
1 tsp	chopped fresh basil	5 mL

1. In ovenproof saucepan, combine tomatoes, oil and thyme. Roast in preheated oven until tomatoes are soft and golden brown, about 30 minutes.

2. Add basil. Transfer to a blender or use an immersion blender in the saucepan. Purée until smooth. Let cool until warm to the touch or transfer to an airtight container and refrigerate for up to 3 days or freeze for up to 1 month.

Nutrients per serving (¼ cup/50 mL)	
Calories 22	Dietary fiber . . . . . . 1.0 g
Protein . . . . 0.8 g	Sodium . . . . 4.2 mg
Total fat . . . . 1.0 g	Calcium . . . . 9.6 mg
Saturated fat. . . . . . 0.1 g	Iron . . . . 0.3 mg
Carbohydrates. . . . . 3.3 g	Vitamin C. . . . . . 11.0 mg

Not just for babies

This should become a staple in your home for everyday use. It makes a great substitute for store-bought ketchups, which contain so much unnecessary sugar, or a delicious spread for sandwiches.

Turnip and Parsnip "Smash"

I first served this great mash at East City Grill in Fort Lauderdale, Fla. It's a wonderful, mild-tasting introduction to the flavor of turnips, and your baby will love it.

Makes about 1 cup (250 mL)

■ ■ ■

Chef Jordan's Tips

When buying turnips to feed to babies, choose those that are relatively small. Turnips can develop a rather strong taste as they grow. Don't confuse turnips with rutabaga, a larger vegetable with a yellowish flesh that is quite a bit more pungent.

Nutrition Tip

While the turnip root is a rich source of many nutrients, including fiber, turnip greens are actually more nutritious. Store the greens separate from the roots but combine them when cooking this purée for a bigger nutritional boost. Cut off and discard the tough stems and wash well. Add the leaves, whole or sliced, to the turnip pot for the last 10 minutes of cooking.

* Potato masher

2 cups	water	500 mL
2 cups	coarsely chopped peeled parsnips	250 mL
1 cup	coarsely chopped peeled white turnip	250 mL

1. In a saucepan, combine water, parsnips and turnip. Bring to a boil over medium heat. Reduce heat to low and simmer until vegetables are soft and most of the water has evaporated, about 20 minutes.

2. Transfer to a blender or use an immersion blender in the saucepan. Purée to your baby's preferred consistency, pulsing for a chunkier consistency. Let cool until warm to the touch or transfer to an airtight container and refrigerate for up to 3 days.

Nutrients per serving (¼ cup/50 mL)

Calories	56	Dietary fiber	3.6 g
Protein	1.0 g	Sodium	29.0 mg
Total fat	0.2 g	Calcium	33.4 mg
Saturated fat	0.0 g	Iron	0.5 mg
Carbohydrates	13.3 g	Vitamin C	17.2 mg

Not just for babies

Remove a serving for Baby and add 1 tbsp (15 mL) chopped chives and ⅓ cup (75 mL) sour cream. This makes an elegant side dish for meat or fish.

Red Cabbage, Fennel and Apple Purée

The combination of cabbage and fennel creates an extraordinary flavor for you and your family.

Makes about 2¼ cups (550 mL)

■ ■ ■

Chef Jordan's Tips

Red cabbage can stain your clothes (a cautionary word to the wise) so wear an apron when making this recipe.

Nutrition Tip

There is more documented research on the anti-cancer properties of the cabbage family, which includes broccoli, cauliflower, kale and Brussels sprouts, than any other vegetable group. The American Cancer Institute recommends including these cruciferous vegetables in your diet on a regular basis to help reduce the risk of cancer. Give your baby every opportunity to acquire a taste for these vegetables because it will likely have long-term benefits for her health.

2 cups	water	500 mL
1 cup	thinly sliced red cabbage	250 mL
¾ cup	coarsely chopped cored Gala apple (about 1)	175 mL
⅓ cup	thinly sliced fresh fennel	75 mL

1. In a saucepan, combine water, cabbage, apple and fennel. Bring to a boil over medium heat. Reduce heat to low and simmer until fennel and cabbage are soft, about 40 minutes.

2. Transfer to a blender or use an immersion blender in the saucepan. Purée to your baby's preferred consistency, pulsing for a chunkier consistency. Let cool until warm to the touch or transfer to an airtight container and refrigerate for up to 3 days or freeze for up to 1 month.

Nutrients per serving (¼ cup/50 mL)	
Calories 20	Dietary fiber . . . . . . 1.5 g
Protein . . . . 0.5 g	Sodium . . . . 12.0 mg
Total fat . . . . 0.1 g	Calcium . . . . 18.8 mg
Saturated fat. . . . . . 0.0 g	Iron . . . . 0.2 mg
Carbohydrates. . . . . 5.0 g	Vitamin C. . . . . . 12.3 mg

Not just for babies

Mom and Dad, this makes a superb accompaniment for roast pork or grilled pork chops. Enjoy.

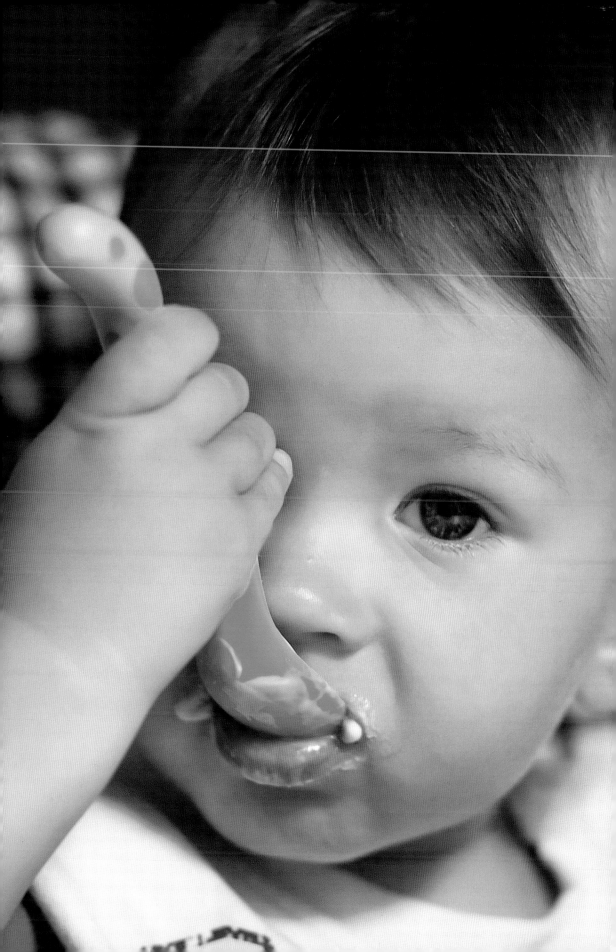

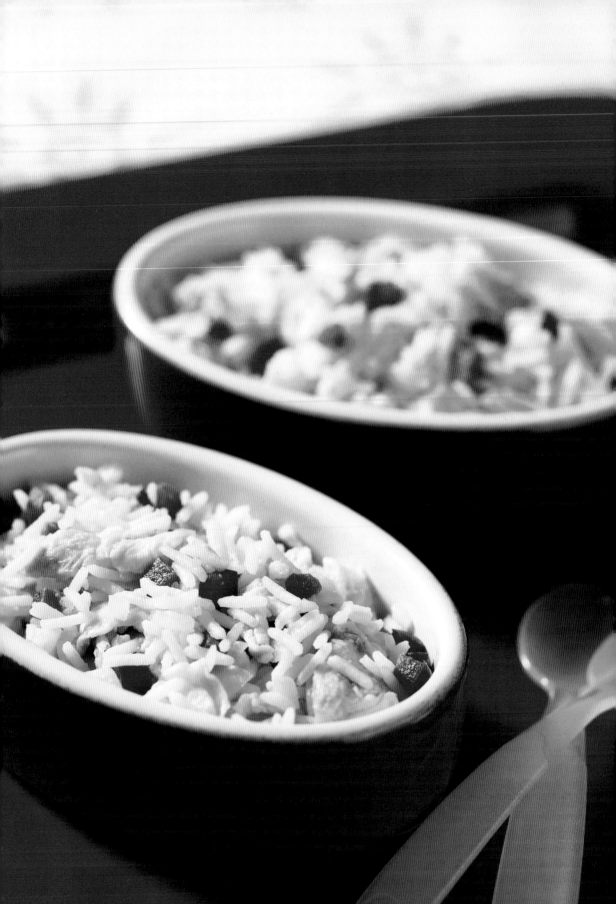

Egg and Sweet Pepper Fried Rice (page 91)

Israeli Couscous with Grated Carrots and Chives (page 144)

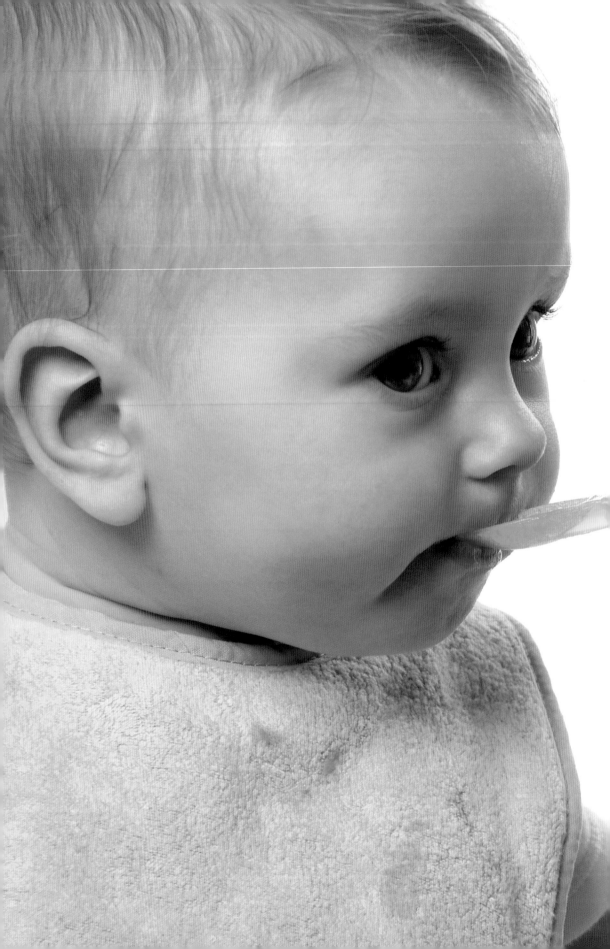

Roasted Onion Soubise

Aside from sugary desserts, this soubise has the sweetest flavor you'll ever taste! For extra flavor, make it using Roasted Chicken Stock (see page 202) instead of water.

Makes about 2 cups (500 mL)

- - -

Chef Jordan's Tips

Classically, a soubise is a purée of onions with a cream-based sauce or straight cream. I choose to cook without creams and heavy sauces. If you're buying the best onions, roasting them should make them taste like heaven. Chicken, beef or vegetable stocks that don't contain salt would all work nicely in place of water.

Nutrition Tip

Onions are a terrific source of prebiotics, which are nondigestible food ingredients. Prebiotics stimulate the growth of friendly bacteria in your baby's large intestine, which supports his immune system and helps prevent harmful bacteria from taking hold.

* Preheat oven to 350°F (180°C)
* Baking sheet

4	sweet onions, such as Vidalia, unpeeled (about 2 large, 1½ lbs/750 g)	4
½ cup	water	125 mL

1. Place onions on baking sheet and roast in preheated oven until soft, about 2 hours. Transfer to a plate and let cool until they can be easily handled. Peel off skins and roughly chop.

2. In a saucepan, combine peeled onions and water. Bring to a boil over medium heat and boil for 5 minutes.

3. Transfer to a blender or use an immersion blender in the saucepan. Purée until smooth. Let cool until warm to the touch or transfer to an airtight container and refrigerate for up to 3 days or freeze up to 1 month.

Nutrients per serving (¼ cup/50 mL)	
Calories 53	Dietary fiber . . . . . . 1.5 g
Protein . . . . 1.3 g	Sodium . . . . 13.7 mg
Total fat . . . . 0.1 g	Calcium . . . . 33.6 mg
Saturated fat. . . . . . 0.0 g	Iron . . . . 0.4 mg
Carbohydrates. . . . 12.5 g	Vitamin C. . . . . . . 7.9 mg

Not just for babies

This purée was always handy when someone requested a pasta dish from one of my kitchens. Its versatility will allow you, after serving Baby, to create a wonderful meal for Mom and Dad. Add it to pasta or serve over roasted chicken.

Potato, Parsnip and Chicken Soup with Chive Parsley "Pistou"

This is one of my favorite and tastiest ways to use up leftover chicken.

Makes about 3½ cups (875 mL)

■ ■ ■

Chef Jordan's Tips

This really is a great way to use up leftover chicken. For added flavor, leave the potato unpeeled and substitute Vegetable Stock (see recipe, page 201) or Roasted Chicken Stock (see recipe, page 202) for the water.

Nutrition Tip

This is an all-in-one meal. You have complete protein from the chicken, complex carbohydrates from the potato and easily digestible fat from the butter. There is an assortment of vitamins and minerals from the parsnips, chives and garlic.

Buy organic potatoes

1 tbsp	unsalted butter	15 mL
1 cup	finely diced baking potato	250 mL
¾ cup	chopped boneless skinless cooked chicken (see Tips, left)	175 mL
½ cup	finely diced peeled parsnip	125 mL
2	cloves garlic, minced	2
3 cups	water (see Tips, left)	750 mL
2 tbsp	Chive Parsley "Pistou" (see recipe, page 99)	25 mL

1. In a saucepan, melt butter over medium heat. Add potato, chicken, parsnip and garlic and cook until potato begins to soften, about 5 minutes. Add water and bring to a boil. Reduce heat and simmer until vegetables are falling apart, about 10 minutes. Remove from heat and stir in pistou.

2. Transfer to a blender or use an immersion blender in the saucepan. Purée to your baby's preferred consistency, pulsing for a chunkier consistency. Let cool until warm to the touch or transfer to an airtight container and refrigerate for up to 3 days.

Nutrients per serving (¼ cup/50 mL)	
Calories 35	Dietary fiber . . . . . . 0.4 g
Protein . . . . 1.3 g	Sodium . . . . 39.1 mg
Total fat . . . . 2.1 g	Calcium . . . . 5.9 mg
Saturated fat. . . . . . 0.7 g	Iron . . . . 0.1 mg
Carbohydrates. . . . . 2.7 g	Vitamin C. . . . . . . 1.9 mg

Not just for babies
Feed some to Baby and enjoy the rest yourself.

Chive Parsley "Pistou"

These days, most of my cuisine is nut-free because of nut allergies in my extended family. This is another spin on a classic, Italian basil pesto, which would normally contain pine nuts. This version, which is more French, contains only the clean flavors of parsley, chives, garlic and olive oil and is wonderful over grain or rice cereals or, as your baby gets older, with noodles and Parmesan cheese. Now would be an ideal occasion to break out that expensive olive oil you've had stashed in the cupboard. Its flavor will shine right through.

Makes about ½ cup (125 mL)

- - -

Chef Jordan's Tips
To create something that resembles the classic Italian basil pesto, spoon off 1 tbsp (15 mL) for Baby, then add ¼ cup (50 mL) pine nuts and ¼ cup (50 mL) Parmesan cheese. You and your significant other will love it. I do not recommend serving nuts to children under 2 years of age.

Nutrition Tip
All green plants contain some amount of chlorophyll, but the greener the vegetable, the more chlorophyll it contains. Parsley's rich green color indicates it is loaded with this nutrient. Chlorophyll fights infections and stimulates new cell growth, two functions that are important for your growing baby.

¾ cup	fresh flat or curly parsley, chopped	175 mL
½ cup	extra virgin olive oil	125 mL
¼ cup	fresh chives, chopped	50 mL
2	cloves garlic, minced	2

1. In a blender, combine parsley, oil, chives and garlic. Purée until smooth. Use immediately or transfer to an airtight container and refrigerate for up to 3 days.

Nutrients per serving (¼ cup/50 mL)	
Calories 547	Dietary fiber . . . . . . 0.9 g
Protein . . . . 1.0 g	Sodium . . . . 13.1 mg
Total fat . . . . 59.4 g	Calcium . . . . 40.7 mg
Saturated fat. . . . . . 8.3 g	Iron . . . . 1.5 mg
Carbohydrates. . . . . 2.6 g	Vitamin C. . . . . . 33.4 mg

Not just for babies
This pistou is the type of "condiment" my wife, Tamar, and I like having in our home. It is so versatile. It can be used for a variety of functions, such as marinating salmon fillets or chicken breast. Or, with the addition of a little champagne vinegar, it can be transformed into a light herb vinaigrette to highlight the smoked salmon you are serving at the next family brunch.

Herb and Spices as Nutrition

Herbs and spices have been used as flavor enhancers for millennia, but now research is showing they also offer a wide range of nutritional benefits. In fact, the USDA reports that ounce for ounce, some herbs and spices have more antioxidant activity than many fresh fruits and vegetables.

Herbs are the green leaves of some plants and, to maximize their healthful properties, it is generally better to use them in their fresh form. Most leafy green herbs — for instance, parsley, thyme and oregano — contain vitamin K, which is important for blood clotting and optimal bone formation. They also have a substantial flavonoid content, which makes them powerful antioxidants. Since fresh is best, why not try growing herbs in the backyard or on the windowsill for a constant fresh supply?

Spices are usually the bark, stem or seeds of a plant that has aromatic properties. However, they have much more to offer than their pleasing scents. For instance, cinnamon is currently being studied for its role in keeping blood sugar under control, which may be of benefit for people with type-2 diabetes, and curcumin, a component of turmeric, has well-documented anti-inflammatory properties. Moreover, there is reason to believe these substances work synergistically. When researchers in India studied the antioxidant ability of individual spices such as cinnamon, pepper and ginger alone and then together, they found the combination produced greater health benefits.

Ratatouille Vegetables

The colors and textures of ratatouille, a vegetable dish that is traditionally French.

**Makes about
1¼ cups (300 mL)**

■ ■ ■

Chef Jordan's Tips

Eggplant skin is easily removed by cutting the eggplant into large discs and laying flat on a cutting board. Trim away the skin using a knife, not a peeler.

Nutrition Tip

What a great way to give your baby the benefit of a whole bunch of vegetables! A recipe like this provides a wide range of vitamins, minerals and phytonutrients that are unlikely to be found in just one vegetable. Ensuring your baby has a varied diet can help prevent a deficiency in any one nutrient.

Buy organic peppers

1 tbsp	unsalted butter	15 mL
¾ cup	finely diced peeled eggplant	175 mL
½ cup	finely diced red bell pepper	125 mL
½ cup	finely diced yellow bell pepper	125 mL
¼ cup	finely diced zucchini	50 mL
¼ cup	finely diced red onion	50 mL
1	sprig fresh thyme	1
⅓ cup	water	75 mL
2	basil leaves, chopped	2

1. In a saucepan, melt butter over medium-low heat. Add eggplant, red and yellow peppers, zucchini, onion and thyme and sauté until vegetables are soft, about 10 minutes. Add water and basil and cook, stirring, until liquid has evaporated, 3 to 5 minutes. Discard thyme.

2. Transfer to a blender or use an immersion blender in the saucepan. Purée to your baby's preferred consistency, pulsing for a chunkier consistency. Let cool until warm to the touch or transfer to an airtight container and refrigerate for up to 3 days.

Nutrients per serving (¼ cup/50 mL)	
Calories 41	Dietary fiber . . . . . . 1.3 g
Protein . . . . 0.8 g	Sodium . . . . 3.9 mg
Total fat . . . . 2.5 g	Calcium . . . . 11.7 mg
Saturated fat. . . . . . 1.5 g	Iron . . . . 0.3 mg
Carbohydrates. . . . . 4.7 g	Vitamin C. . . . . . 52.8 mg

> ### Not just for babies
> Toss this with cubed rare yellowfin tuna and garnish with a few chopped chives.

Sautéed Chard with Apples

The addition of apples makes it much easier to introduce nutrient-dense leafy greens to your baby. The fruit's inherent sweetness complements the flavor very well.

Makes about 1¼ cups (300 mL)

≡ ≡ ≡

Chef Jordan's Tips
Always take care when adding hot liquids to a blender. Fill the container no more than half full or allow to cool before blending.

Nutrition Tip
Chard's combination of phytochemicals (particularly anthocyans), vitamins, minerals, fiber and chlorophyll make it an incredibly potent anti-cancer food. By starting your baby on Swiss chard early, you are providing him with lifelong health benefits.

Buy organic apples

1 tbsp	unsalted butter	15 mL
½ cup	finely diced cored peeled Granny Smith apple	125 mL
⅓ cup	finely diced sweet onion	75 mL
3 cups	chopped Swiss chard	750 mL
¾ cup	water	175 mL

1. In a saucepan, melt butter over medium heat. Add apple and onion and sauté until onion is translucent, about 3 minutes. Add chard and sauté until wilted, 3 to 4 minutes. Add water and bring to a boil. Reduce heat to low and simmer until most of the liquid has evaporated, about 15 minutes.

2. Transfer to a blender or use an immersion blender in the saucepan. Purée to your baby's preferred consistency, pulsing for a chunkier consistency. Let cool until warm to the touch or transfer to an airtight container and refrigerate for up to 3 days.

Nutrients per serving (¼ cup/50 mL)	
Calories 34	Dietary fiber . . . . . . 0.7 g
Protein . . . . 0.6 g	Sodium . . . . 47.8 mg
Total fat . . . . 2.4 g	Calcium . . . . 15.7 mg
Saturated fat. . . . . . 1.5 g	Iron . . . . 0.4 mg
Carbohydrates. . . . . 3.2 g	Vitamin C. . . . . . . 7.7 mg

Not just for babies
I once asked NBA great Charles Oakley about the his mother's greens. "Man, you got to always use apples when cooking your greens," he said. I now cook greens with apples, any apples. The combination belongs together, and it's not just for babies.

Fresh Soy Bean Hummus

This is a particularly nutritious variation on one of my favorite purées. Hummus is my spread of choice. I love it on everything, from chicken breast to bread. Your family will, too.

**Makes about
2 cups (500 mL)**

■ ■ ■

Chef Jordan's Tips
Fresh or frozen soy beans are widely available in grocery chains, typically in the health/organic freezer section. In their absence, green peas are an excellent substitute.

Nutrition Tip
The numerous health-promoting benefits of soy beans include the fact that they are a complete protein source, high in fiber, and contain essential fatty acids as well as phytonutrients such as phytosterols and isoflavones. The benefits of essential fats are immediate for your baby because they are crucial for good brain development.

2 cups	cooked chickpeas, drained and rinsed (see page 77)	500 mL
1 cup	water	250 mL
½ cup	fresh or frozen soy beans (edamame)	125 mL
2	cloves garlic	2

1. In a saucepan, combine chickpeas, water, soy beans and garlic. Bring to a boil over medium heat, cover and simmer until soy beans are soft, about 3 minutes.
2. Transfer to a blender or use an immersion blender in the saucepan. Purée until smooth. Let cool to room temperature or transfer to an airtight container and refrigerate for up to 3 days.

Nutrients per serving (¼ cup/50 mL)	
Calories 76	Dietary fiber . . . . . . 2.7 g
Protein . . . . 5.2 g	Sodium . . . . . . 173.6 mg
Total fat . . . . 1.9 g	Calcium . . . . 55.6 mg
Saturated fat. . . . . . 0.1 g	Iron . . . . 1.3 mg
Carbohydrates. . . . 10.1 g	Vitamin C. . . . . . . 5.1 mg

Not just for babies
This purée, as is, makes an excellent addition to any adult meal. Serve it over flatbread as an appetizer if you're enjoying a glass of wine before dinner.

White Bean and Fennel Purée

This purée is an awesome baby food, soup or dip for vegetables when those unexpected guests drop in. This recipe yields enough for your baby and you to enjoy.

Makes about 1¾ cups (425 mL)

■ ■ ■

Chef Jordan's Tips

In many of the establishments I've worked in we welcomed our guests with an "amuse bouche." One of my favorites was a small piece of braised lamb set on a spoonful of this purée. This flavor combination is so good, some of the guests requested a full-size serving for their meal.

Nutrition Tip

One of the challenges of a vegetarian diet is ensuring that it contains enough protein. Legumes (dried beans and lentils) are one of the best vegetarian sources of protein, even though they don't contain all eight essential amino acids. However, this purée can be combined with one of our grain recipes, such as brown rice or quinoa, to provide your baby with the complete range of amino acids.

1 cup	soaked white beans, such as navy or cannellini (see page 77)	250 mL
4 cups	water	1 L
1¼ cups	coarsely chopped fresh fennel	300 mL

1. In a saucepan, combine beans, water and fennel. Bring to a boil over medium heat. Reduce heat to low and simmer until beans are soft, about 75 minutes.

2. Transfer to a blender or use an immersion blender in the saucepan. Purée to your baby's preferred consistency, pulsing for a chunkier consistency. Let cool until warm to the touch or transfer to an airtight container and refrigerate for up to 3 days or freeze for up to 1 month.

Nutrients per serving (¼ cup/50 mL)

Calories 44	Dietary fiber ...... 3.5 g
Protein .... 2.5 g	Sodium .... 17.1 mg
Total fat .... 0.2 g	Calcium .... 34.3 mg
Saturated fat...... 0.0 g	Iron .... 0.8 mg
Carbohydrates..... 8.6 g	Vitamin C....... 3.2 mg

Not just for babies

I love this purée — it's versatile enough to feed your baby a uniquely flavored purée and hearty enough for Mom and Dad to have as a dip for vegetables as a light hors d'oeuvre, or as a side dish under your lamb, beef, chicken or fish.

Using Canned Beans

Although canned beans are more convenient, most are problematic, even for adults, because they are loaded with sodium. If you are using canned beans, be sure to rinse them very well to remove as much of the added salt as possible.

Sodium is a necessary mineral in the body and is found in many foods, including vegetables and breast milk, but no one needs the excessive amounts of sodium usually added to canned foods. Too much sodium from the wrong sources can contribute to a variety of health problems, from high blood pressure to heart disease. A few companies are producing canned beans, usually organic, with no salt added. These may be seasoned with seaweed, which is fine for your baby to have. Seaweed does contain sodium, but in acceptable amounts. It also contains beneficial minerals like iodine. Your thyroid gland, which regulates your body's metabolism, won't function at its best without an adequate supply of iodine.

Whether you are using canned beans or soaking your own, beans (and other legumes, such as lentils) are an important part of a healthful diet. We recommend eating them at least three times a week. Legumes are a good source of protein, fiber and minerals such as calcium and iron. Eating them regularly can help protect against type-2 diabetes, among other diseases. They also promote good bowel health.

Oven-Roasted Chicken with Dried Apricots

My mother-in-law introduced me to this flavor combination. She's not the greatest cook in the world (I will be removing this page from her copy of this book), so she will be surprised to hear that I learned something culinary from her. Thank you, Lee!

Makes about
1½ cups (375 mL)

■ ■ ■

Chef Jordan's Tips

People are always staring at me in the grocery store because they see me smelling every last piece of fruit I purchase to ensure that my family has the best and freshest available. I've always chosen fruit with my nose first because if it smells like a great apricot it should taste like one, too. After the fruit passes the smell test, try to choose an apricot that is neither too firm nor too soft. The flesh should spring back if poked lightly with your finger.

- Preheat oven to 350°F (180°C)
- Ovenproof skillet

8 oz	bone-in skin-on chicken thighs (2 thighs)	250 g
5	fresh apricots, pitted (about 6 oz/175 g)	5
½ cup	water	125 mL

1. In ovenproof skillet, combine chicken, apricots and water. Roast in a preheated oven until chicken is golden brown and juices run clear when pierced, 35 to 40 minutes. Let cool until chicken can be easily handled. Remove skin and remove meat from the bone, discarding skin and bones.

2. Transfer chicken and apricots to a blender or to a cup or bowl and use an immersion blender. Purée to your baby's preferred consistency, pulsing for a chunkier consistency. Serve immediately or transfer to an airtight container and refrigerate for up to 3 days.

Nutrients per serving (¼ cup/50 mL)	
Calories 71	Dietary fiber . . . . . . 0.6 g
Protein . . . . 5.9 g	Sodium . . . . 25.0 mg
Total fat . . . . 3.8 g	Calcium . . . . 7.5 mg
Saturated fat. . . . . . 1.1 g	Iron . . . . 0.4 mg
Carbohydrates. . . . . 3.2 g	Vitamin C. . . . . . . 3.7 mg

Not just for babies

Double this recipe and spoon off a serving for your baby. Remove the remainder of the chicken from the bone, leaving the apricots whole and serve (without puréeing, of course) over couscous. It's an excellent combination for lunch or dinner.

Fresh apricots are extremely perishable and available seasonally in North America in June and July. Although fresh apricots are best, dried can be substituted in this recipe. Use about 10 dried apricots to replace this quantity of fresh.

Nutrition Tip

Free-range poultry has the benefits of having more room to roam, which can affect the taste and quality of the meat. It may be lower in fat and have a richer taste. If it's naturally raised, free-range chicken will also be antibiotic- and hormone-free and far less likely to be infected with salmonella than a factory bird. Choose organic/naturally raised poultry when you can.

Chicken with Roasted Butternut Squash and Leeks

I love how the sweetness of the leeks complements the chicken and squash.

Makes about 1½ cups (375 mL)

■ ■ ■

Chef Jordan's Tips

Dark meat is my preference when cooking for babies because of the higher fat content but in a pinch, I wouldn't hesitate to use a chicken breast if it was all that was available.

Nutrition Tip

When your baby is this age, you can offer him poultry or other protein sources such as legumes, egg yolks, tofu or meat a couple of times a day. The vegetables in this recipe add a variety of vitamins, minerals and phytonutrients, making it a well-rounded meal that will promote growth and development.

1 tbsp	unsalted butter	15 mL
¾ cup	diced and peeled butternut squash	175 mL
1	diced boneless, skinless chicken thigh (about 4 oz/125 g)	1
½ cup	chopped leeks, white part only	125 mL
1 cup	water	250 mL

1. In a saucepan, over medium heat, melt butter. Add squash and sauté until golden, about 5 minutes. Add chicken and leeks and sauté until leeks are wilted, about 2 minutes. Add water and bring to a boil. Reduce heat to low and simmer until chicken is cooked through, about 5 minutes.

2. Transfer to a blender or use an immersion blender in the saucepan. Purée to your baby's preferred consistency, pulsing for a chunkier consistency. Let cool until warm to the touch or transfer to an airtight container and refrigerate for up to 3 days.

Nutrients per serving (¼ cup/50 mL)	
Calories 48	Dietary fiber . . . . . . 0.7 g
Protein . . . . 2.7 g	Sodium . . . . 14.0 mg
Total fat . . . . 2.4 g	Calcium . . . . 21.7 mg
Saturated fat. . . . . . 1.3 g	Iron . . . . 0.5 mg
Carbohydrates. . . . . 4.5 g	Vitamin C. . . . . . . 7.2 mg

Not just for babies

Purée ½ cup (125 mL) for Baby. The balance is a stew for Mom and Dad. Add 1 cup (250 mL) whole milk and 2 tbsp (25 mL) Chive Parsley "Pistou" (page 99) and bring to a boil.

Pork Tenderloin and Peaches

If you enjoy barbecue, try this recipe. You'll think you're in the Deep South!

Makes about 1¼ cups (300 mL)

■ ■ ■

Chef Jordan's Tips

Beurre noisette is the French term for brown butter, a versatile ingredient used in sauces, vinaigrettes or pan searing. In this case, browning the butter and searing the pork develops a crisp, golden brown outside that creates a flavor profile typically reserved for 5-star meals.

Nutrition Tip

Pork is the highest meat source of thiamin (vitamin B_3), which is one of the many B-complex vitamins necessary for the optimal use of all foods in your baby's body. It is also essential for the growth and repair of nerve and muscle tissue.

1 tsp	unsalted butter	5 mL
1 cup	coarsely chopped sweet onions	250 mL
1	peach, pitted and sliced	1
4 oz	pork tenderloin, sliced into 4 medallions	125 g
1 cup	water	250 mL

1. In a saucepan, melt butter over high heat until turning a slight hazelnut-brown color, about 1 minute (see Tips, left). Add onions, peach and pork and sauté until pork is golden brown, about 5 minutes. Add water and bring to a boil. Reduce heat and simmer until water has reduced by half, about 7 minutes.

2. Transfer to a blender or use an immersion blender in the saucepan. Purée to your baby's preferred consistency, pulsing for a chunkier consistency. Let cool until warm to the touch or transfer to an airtight container and refrigerate for up to 3 days.

Nutrients per serving (¼ cup/50 mL)	
Calories 62	Dietary fiber . . . . . . 0.6 g
Protein . . . . 5.8 g	Sodium . . . . 14.5 mg
Total fat . . . . 2.4 g	Calcium . . . . 6.9 mg
Saturated fat. . . . . . 1.0 g	Iron . . . . 0.4 mg
Carbohydrates. . . . . 4.4 g	Vitamin C. . . . . . . 2.9 mg

Not just for babies

This recipe makes an awesome wonton stuffing. Place a small amount of the purée in the middle of the wonton wrapper and seal. Cook wontons in a large pot of water, just at the boil, until they rise to the surface. Remove with a slotted spoon.

Beef Tenderloin and Dates

This is a slightly sweet and very enjoyable meat purée. Babies will love it and, Mom and Dad, you'll be tempted to eat it all.

Makes about 1¼ cups (300 mL)

▪ ▪ ▪

Chef Jordan's Tips

Dates are quite easy to find in grocery stores. In this recipe, they impart a unique flavor profile but could easily be replaced by an equal quantity of prunes, dried apricots or dried peaches.

Nutrition Tip

Dates contain easily digestible carbohydrates along with considerable amounts of important energy-promoting B vitamins. Combined with the protein in the beef, this recipe provides long-lasting energy to fuel your active baby.

1 tsp	unsalted butter	5 mL
⅓ cup	diced beef tenderloin	75 mL
1¼ cups	water	300 mL
¼ cup	dates, pitted	50 mL

1. In a saucepan, over medium heat, melt butter. Add beef and cook, stirring, until browned, about 3 minutes. Add water and dates and bring to a boil. Cook until liquid is reduced by half, 5 to 6 minutes.

2. Transfer to a blender or use an immersion blender in the saucepan. Purée to your baby's preferred consistency, pulsing for a chunkier consistency. Let cool until warm to the touch or transfer to an airtight container and refrigerate for up to 3 days or freeze for up to 1 month.

Nutrients per serving (¼ cup/50 mL)			
Calories	46	Dietary fiber	0.6 g
Protein	3.0 g	Sodium	9.0 mg
Total fat	1.3 g	Calcium	6.0 mg
Saturated fat	0.7 g	Iron	0.4 mg
Carbohydrates	6.4 g	Vitamin C	0.0 mg

Not just for babies

Believe it or not, this would make an excellent accompaniment to a grilled steak individually served on a plate or sliced on a platter. I always love my meats, cooked to perfection of course, to be displayed with the sauce underneath as opposed to draped overtop; it looks nicer and maintains that beautiful sheen grilled meat has once rested. To garnish, I suggest some finely diced dates. I'm hungry thinking about it.

Lamb with Parsnips and Dried Cranberries

Your baby will love the flavor combination of cranberries and lamb.

Makes about 1¼ cups (300 mL)

- - -

Chef Jordan's Tips

As this recipe cooks quite quickly, I suggest using a lean and tender cut of meat such as the loin.

Nutrition Tip

As well as being a rich source of many minerals, meat is our primary source of the vitamin B_{12}, which is very important to keep your nervous system functioning well. However, meat doesn't contain any fiber. The parsnips and cranberries in this recipe provide that nutrient, which among its many benefits helps to keep your baby from becoming constipated.

1 tsp	unsalted butter	5 mL
½ cup	finely diced parsnip	125 mL
¼ cup	finely diced lamb (about 2 oz/60 g), (see Tips, left)	50 mL
2 tbsp	dried cranberries	25 mL
1 cup	water	250 mL

1. In a saucepan, over medium heat, melt butter. Add parsnip, lamb and cranberries and sauté until meat begins to brown, about 3 minutes. Add water and bring to a boil. Reduce heat to low and simmer until parsnip is soft, about 8 minutes.

2. Transfer to a blender or use an immersion blender in the saucepan. Purée to your baby's preferred consistency, pulsing for a chunkier consistency. Let cool until warm to the touch or transfer to an airtight container and refrigerate for up to 3 days or freeze for up to 1 month.

Nutrients per serving (¼ cup/50 mL)	
Calories 41	Dietary fiber . . . . . . 0.8 g
Protein . . . . 2.4 g	Sodium . . . . 10.1 mg
Total fat . . . . 1.4 g	Calcium . . . . 7.5 mg
Saturated fat. . . . . 0.7 g	Iron . . . . 0.3 mg
Carbohydrates. . . . 4.9 g	Vitamin C. . . . . . . 2.3 mg

Not Just for Babies

Sorry, Mom and Dad. This is one of those rare dishes that does just work for Baby.

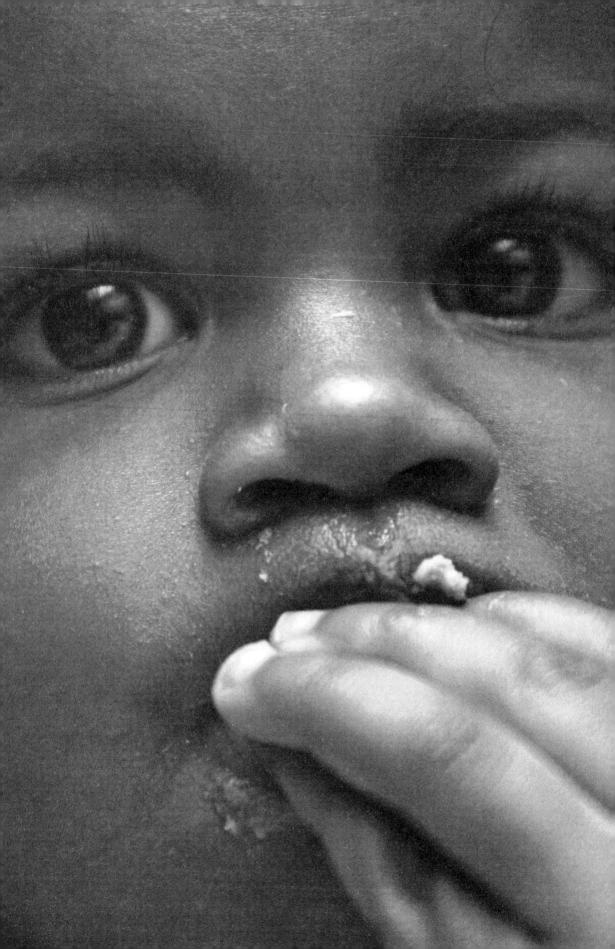

Food for Toddlers
(12 Months +)

Introduction 114

Fruit
Strawberries with Granny Smith
    Apples 116
Nectarine and Orange Compote . . . 117
Apple and Strawberry Compote . . . 118
Warm Pineapple with Cottage
    Cheese and Basil 119
Roasted Summer Fruit. 120
Roasted Summer Fruit Smoothie . . . 121
Citrus Fruit Salad with Fresh Basil . . 122
Papaya and Coconut Milk Purée . . . 123

Vegetables
Oven-Roasted Artichokes 124
Quick Mushroom Soup 126
Corn and Chickpea Chowder 127
Asparagus and Roasted Tomato . . . 128
Fennel and Orange Sauté 130
"Smashed" Baby Potatoes 131
Crispy Potato Galette 132
Broccoli, Potato and Spinach Pie . . . 133
Grilled Asparagus with
    Three Cheeses. 134
Red Potato Salad with Cheddar
    Cheese and Boiled Eggs 135
Best-Ever Barbecued Corn 136
Oven-Roasted Cauliflower
    with Fresh Herbs. 137

Grains
Jonah's "Mac and Cheese". 138
Basic Pearled Barley 139

Warm Barley with Fresh Herbs
    and Parmesan Cheese. 140
Millet and Cauliflower with
    Fresh Oregano 141
Creamy Brown Rice and
    Fresh Basil 142
Soft Polenta with Cheddar Cheese
    and Broccoli Florets. 143
Israeli Couscous with Grated
    Carrots and Chives 144
Jasmine Rice with Butternut
    Squash and Saffron. 145
Whole-Grain Oat Crêpes
    with Warm Bananas 146
French Toast with Fresh Peaches
    and Peachy Maple Syrup 148

Fish
World's Best "Fish Sticks". 150
Alaskan Halibut en Papillote. 152
Salmon, Potato and Cauliflower . . . 154
Pacific Salmon Cakes 155

Meat
Classic Beef and Barley Stew 156
Fennel and Apple-Stuffed
    Pork Chops. 158
Pork with Red Cabbage 160
Fresh Herb-Crusted Veal Chops. . . . 161
Chicken with Caramelized Apples . . 162
Onion Soup with Cornish Hen. 163
Gramma Jean's Turkey Meatloaf . . . 164
Oven-Roasted Duck Confit
    with Fresh Thyme 166
Red Cabbage with Duck Confit. . . . 167

Introduction

The changes that happen around the time your baby celebrates his first birthday are quite exciting. All the crawling, "scooting" and walking he is likely doing increases his need for energy in the form of nutrient-dense calories. The problem is, toddlers are so busy exploring, they may not want to sit still long enough to eat. This may mean that you need to feed your toddler more frequently — from four to six times a day, in addition to his milk intake. Appropriate finger foods may be one way to meet this increased demand.

When first introducing finger foods, steamed vegetables or soft fruits, such as tiny broccoli trees or bits of ripe banana, are a good choice because he is familiar with the tastes from the purées he enjoyed as early foods. Also, these foods are easy to pick up and eat. As his dexterity increases and he progresses to being able to tolerate and enjoy foods with more texture, he will be able to expand his range and enjoy foods such as thin strips of raw cucumber and red pepper or grated carrots and thin slices of apple. The recipes in this chapter offer exciting new tastes, many of which can be enjoyed by the whole family. They can be mashed or cut to suit your child's preferences.

Feeding a toddler has its challenges, especially when he makes it clear he is not going to eat a particular food today. It is important to stick with the habits you have already established — continue to offer a variety of vegetables, fruit, protein and whole grains. It may take a dozen or two attempts to get your child to try something new, but when he does, he may discover a new favorite. Food dislikes are often learned behavior, so be aware of your food habits, too. Just because you don't like something doesn't mean you shouldn't prepare it for your child. Who knows, maybe it will even taste better to you this time around.

Instead of being too focused on the amount of food your toddler is eating at one sitting, look at his food intake over several days. Children's appetites vary depending on their rate of growth, their surroundings and whether they are tired. It is important for you to remain patient and flexible. You need to be ready to address your child's changing preferences while continuing to offer a variety of nutritious foods.

At this age, snacks (see Chapter 4) become important, as they provide your toddler with energy between meals and may help prevent him from becoming overly hungry or too cranky to eat a proper meal. Choose wisely and don't rely on snacks that contain sugar and/or processed grains. Prepare soft fruits and vegetables in advance so your toddler gets healthy whole foods even when you're out and about.

When you're on the go, it's particularly easy to succumb to the temptation of prepared foods because they are so convenient. Soft fruits, vegetables, plain rice cakes, strips of whole grain bread or pita and small cubes of cheese can be prepared in advance and stored in snack-sized containers that are ready to go. As valuable as snacks are, sticking to a regular meal pattern is also important because toddlers need routine. A regular schedule will encourage good eating habits and will predispose your toddler to enjoy the socializing that takes place when sharing a nutritious meal with his family.

Strawberries with Granny Smith Apples

This recipe is unlike most foods for baby as the apple is left raw, lending unique flavor and texture. Your baby will love this for breakfast, or as a dessert or an afternoon snack.

**Makes about
1 cup (250 mL)**

- - -

Chef Jordan's Tips
In season, substitute any berry you like. If using raspberries or blackberries, cook for about 10 minutes, then strain to get rid of the bitter seeds. Add the apples and mash.

Nutrition Tip
Fresh apples are on almost every list of super foods. After his first birthday, your baby will start eating bits and pieces of cut-up apple. To reduce the amount of "rusting" (when the apple turns brown or oxidizes) dip the pieces in a solution of lemon juice and water. For one apple, use about 3 cups (750 mL) of water and ¼ cup (50 mL) fresh lemon juice.

Buy organic apples

¾ cup	whole strawberries, stems removed	175 mL
¾ cup	water	175 mL
⅔ cup	finely chopped cored Granny Smith apples	150 mL

1. In a saucepan, combine strawberries and water. Bring to a boil over high heat. Reduce heat to low and simmer until strawberries are soft and water has reduced by half, about 8 minutes. Remove from heat, add apple and mash or cut to desired consistency.

2. Let cool until warm to the touch or transfer to an airtight container and refrigerate for up to 3 days or freeze for up to 1 month.

Nutrients per serving (½ cup/125 mL)	
Calories 61	Dietary fiber . . . . . . 3.2 g
Protein . . . . 0.8 g	Sodium . . . . 4.3 mg
Total fat . . . . 0.3 g	Calcium . . . . 20.4 mg
Saturated fat. . . . . . 0.0 g	Iron . . . . 0.5 mg
Carbohydrates. . . . 16.0 g	Vitamin C. . . . . . 55.2 mg

Not just for babies
Mom and Dad, this recipe makes an excellent spread. Try it on your toast in the morning.

Nectarine and Orange Compote

The sweetness of this compote makes an excellent complement to a savory dinner of beef, pork or chicken, but it can also top hot cereal or be served on its own as a dessert.

**Makes about
1¼ cups (300 mL)**

▪ ▪ ▪

Chef Jordan's Tips
Although I suggest creating this dish with citrus fruit segments, I prefer the slightly more labor intensive version of "supremes," which means to remove the skin, pith and membranes of a citrus fruit and separate its wedges. Supremes are much more delicate and easier for children to eat.

Nutrition Tip
The orange and nectarine in this recipe provide healthy doses of vitamin C and enough sweetness so the compote can be used as a dessert.

Buy organic nectarines

1 tsp	unsalted butter	5 mL
1½ cups	diced pitted nectarines	375 mL
½ cup	orange segments (see Tips, left)	250 mL
1	stick cinnamon (about 2 inches/5 cm long)	1

1. In a saucepan, melt butter over medium-low heat. Add nectarines, orange segments and cinnamon stick and sauté until nectarines are soft while still maintaining their shape, about 5 minutes. Let cool until warm to the touch or transfer to an airtight container and refrigerate for up to 3 days. Discard cinnamon stick before serving.

Nutrients per serving (½ cup/125 mL)	
Calories 112	Dietary fiber . . . . . . 3.4 g
Protein . . . . 2.1 g	Sodium . . . . 22.3 mg
Total fat . . . . 3.1 g	Calcium . . . . 37.4 mg
Saturated fat. . . . . . 1.2 g	Iron . . . . 0.5 mg
Carbohydrates. . . . 21.2 g	Vitamin C. . . . . . 45.2 mg

Not just for babies
I love to pair certain foodstuffs with fruits — duck and pork specifically. Just the thought of a duck breast with very crisp skin, sliced thinly, served on a platter beside this compote makes my mouth water.

Apple and Strawberry Compote

Now that Jonah attends junior kindergarten, instead of packing store-bought, packaged fruit mixes, which are loaded with unwanted sugar, in his lunch, I send him to school with this, and guess what? All the other kids want to trade with him. Can you blame them?

Makes about 1¼ cups (300 mL)

■ ■ ■

Chef Jordan's Tips

I encourage you to experiment with vinegars as often as you can because they can be used to season dishes other than salad dressings, such as this delicious compote.

Nutrition Tip

Eating is as much about the social circumstances in which food is consumed as it is about the food itself. Being rushed, stressed and not fully present at family meals can actually impair healthy digestion. Create an environment where an easy pace, laughter and gentle discussion are the guests that join you and your little one at the table.

Buy organic apples

1 tsp	unsalted butter	5 mL
2 cups	diced cored peeled apples	500 mL
½ cup	diced strawberries	125 mL
½ tsp	white wine vinegar	2 mL

1. In a saucepan, melt butter over medium-low heat. Add apples and strawberries and sauté until strawberries have virtually disintegrated, about 10 minutes. Remove from heat and stir in vinegar. Let cool until warm to the touch or transfer to an airtight container and refrigerate for up to 3 days.

Nutrients per serving (½ cup/125 mL)

Calories	68	Dietary fiber	1.8 g
Protein	0.5 g	Sodium	0.5 mg
Total fat	1.8 g	Calcium	10.0 mg
Saturated fat	1.0 g	Iron	0.2 mg
Carbohydrates	14.2 g	Vitamin C	21.6 mg

Not just for babies

This compote makes a wonderful garnish for warm apple pie.

Warm Pineapple with Cottage Cheese and Basil

Growing up, I remember eating something that resembled this but my mother made hers using canned pineapple. Really, Mom, there's nothing like the taste of warm, fresh pineapple.

Makes about 3½ cups (875 mL)

■ ■ ■

Chef Jordan's Tips

Although it's not my preference, many stores sell peeled sliced pineapple. Use it here solely for the purpose of convenience.

Nutrition Tip

Pineapple contains a unique extract called bromelain that is a protein-digesting enzyme. This means it is an excellent digestive aid. The pineapple in this recipe will help your baby digest the protein-rich cottage cheese.

½ cup	water	125 mL
2 cups	diced fresh pineapple (about 12 oz/375 g)	500 mL
1 tsp	chopped basil leaves	5 mL
2 cups	full-fat cottage cheese	500 mL

1. In a saucepan, bring water to a boil over high heat. Add pineapple. Reduce heat to medium-low and simmer until water has fully evaporated and pineapple is caramelized, about 15 minutes. Stir in basil. Mash or cut to desired consistency. Let cool to room temperature or transfer to an airtight container and refrigerate for up to 3 days.

2. Serve over cottage cheese.

Nutrients per serving (½ cup/125 mL)	
Calories 90	Dietary fiber . . . . . . 0.6 g
Protein . . . . 7.7 g	Sodium . . . . . . 246.7 mg
Total fat . . . . 2.9 g	Calcium . . . . 63.6 mg
Saturated fat. . . . . . 1.7 g	Iron . . . . 0.1 mg
Carbohydrates. . . . . 8.5 g	Vitamin C. . . . . . 16.1 mg

Not just for babies

I have fond memories of eating "cottage cheese and pineapple" with my parents and siblings for breakfast, lunch or dinner. It was the "go-to" meal whenever one of us was rushing off to something like hockey practice or dance lessons.

Roasted Summer Fruit

This recipe works for virtually any fruit and can be served with breakfast, lunch and dinner.

Makes about 4 cups (1 L)

∎ ∎ ∎

Chef Jordan's Tips

The combination of the natural sugars in the fruit with brown sugar results in a very rich caramel. The key to caramelization is patience but it's really worth the wait!

In winter substitute apples for the peaches or cranberries or frozen berries for the berries.

Nutrition Tip

We recommend choosing organic peaches and strawberries for this recipe since conventionally grown peaches and strawberries are among the foods on which pesticide residues have been most frequently found.

- Preheat oven to 300°F (150°C)
- Baking dish, lightly greased
- Potato masher, optional

2	peaches, pitted	2
1½ cups	fresh raspberries	375 mL
1½ cups	fresh blueberries	375 mL
1½ cups	whole strawberries, stems removed	375 mL
2	plums, pitted	2
2 tbsp	evaporated cane juice sugar or packed brown sugar	25 mL

1. In prepared baking dish, combine peaches, raspberries, blueberries, strawberries, plums and sugar, stirring until fruit is evenly coated with sugar.

2. Roast in preheated oven until fruit is soft and nicely caramelized (see Tips, left), about 1 hour. Mash or cut to desired consistency. Let cool until warm to the touch or transfer to an airtight container and refrigerate for up to 3 days or freeze for up to 1 month.

Nutrients per serving (½ cup/125 mL)	
Calories 65	Dietary fiber . . . . . . 2.1 g
Protein . . . . 1.0 g	Sodium . . . . 0.6 mg
Total fat . . . . 0.2 g	Calcium . . . . 10.5 mg
Saturated fat. . . . . . 0.0 g	Iron . . . . 0.3 mg
Carbohydrates. . . . 17.3 g	Vitamin C. . . . . . 27.6 mg

Not just for babies
Serve this with pancakes in the morning, with a touch of whipped cream for an afternoon snack or as a condiment with seared pork tenderloin.

Roasted Summer Fruit Smoothie

What an excellent, healthy treat for your children and you — enjoy!

**Makes about
5 cups (1.25 L)**

■ ■ ■

Chef Jordan's Tips

Vanilla ice cream, sour cream or whipping (35%) cream all make excellent additions or substitutions for yogurt in this recipe.

Nutrition Tip

To ensure optimum nutrition for your baby, supplement this recipe with a good protein powder and healthy oils. One scoop of protein powder (ask your local health food store for a good recommendation for your baby) and a teaspoon (5 mL) or so of hemp or flax seed oil, which provide essential omega-3 fats, will optimize the ratio among carbohydrates, proteins and fats — the three macronutrients your baby needs for growth.

4 cups	Roasted Summer Fruit (see recipe, page 120)	1 L
½ cup	full-fat yogurt	125 mL
½ cup	ice cubes	125 mL
1 tbsp	chopped fresh mint	15 mL

1. In a blender, combine fruit, yogurt, ice cubes and mint. Purée until smooth. Serve immediately.

Nutrients per serving (½ cup/125 mL)

Calories 37	Dietary fiber . . . . . . 1.7 g
Protein . . . . 1.0 g	Sodium . . . . 7.8 mg
Total fat . . . . 0.4 g	Calcium . . . . 31.1 mg
Saturated fat. . . . . . 0.3 g	Iron . . . . 1.1 mg
Carbohydrates. . . . . 7.2 g	Vitamin C. . . . . . 12.1 mg

Not just for babies

I owe this simple recipe to my sister-in-law Michelle. Previously, I always worked out on an empty stomach to avoid getting heartburn. Michelle introduced me to a fresh fruit smoothie one glorious summer day before a marathon walk and I felt great! Now, when they are in season, I'll buy a surplus of my favorite fruits, roast them and freeze them. That way I don't even need ice. I just combine all the ingredients in a blender and purée, then head off for a workout, heartburn free!

Citrus Fruit Salad with Fresh Basil

This is a very refreshing fruit salad not only for Baby but also for the rest of the family. We love eating this right from the fridge on hot summer days.

Makes about 2½ cups (625 mL)

■ ■ ■

Chef Jordan's Tips

Although citrus fruit segments will work in this dish, I prefer to make "supremes," which are are much more delicate and easier for children to eat. Separate citrus fruit into wedges and remove the skin, pith and membrane.

Nutrition Tip

Citrus fruits and their skins are loaded with antioxidants that work from the inside out, protecting your baby's delicate skin from premature development of skin damage. The skins contain hyaluronic acid (a component of connective tissue), which is important in the body for tissue repair. Hyaluronic acid has been called "the key to the fountain of youth."

1⅔ cups	grapefruit segments (see Tips, left)	400 mL
1 tsp	grated orange zest	5 mL
1 cup	orange segments	250 mL
½ cup	clementine segments	125 mL
¼ cup	freshly squeezed lemon juice	50 mL
1 tbsp	pure maple syrup	15 mL
1 tsp	chopped basil leaves	5 mL

1. In a bowl, combine grapefruit segments, orange zest and segments, clementine segments, lemon juice, syrup and basil. Cover and refrigerate overnight or for up to 3 days.

Nutrients per serving (½ cup/125 mL)

Calories 65	Dietary fiber . . . . . . 2.2 g
Protein . . . . 1.0 g	Sodium . . . . 0.9 mg
Total fat . . . . 0.2 g	Calcium . . . . 35.2 mg
Saturated fat. . . . . . 0.0 g	Iron . . . . 0.2 mg
Carbohydrates. . . . 16.8 g	Vitamin C. . . . . . 56.1 mg

Not just for babies

Serve this with breakfast muesli or over plain yogurt or, like the Wagman family, straight from the fridge.

Papaya and Coconut Milk Purée

Early in my career, I had the opportunity to cook briefly with the Hawaiian chef, Sam Choy. In our few days together I developed a great appreciation for Hawaiian flavors, which I've tried to capture in this recipe.

Makes about 2½ cups (625 mL)

- - -

Chef Jordan's Tips
When tomatoes are in season, they make an excellent alternative or complement to some of the papaya in the recipe.

Nutrition Tip
Coconut milk, not to be confused with coconut water (found sitting inside the fruit) is made from soaked grated coconut flesh. The fat content of coconut is very high in saturated fat, which is fine for your baby. Coconut oil appears to have many healthful properties. For instance, it is high in lauric acid, which apparently has antibacterial and antifungal properties.

2 cups	chopped peeled papaya	500 mL
1 cup	water	250 mL
½ cup	unsweetened coconut milk	125 mL
½ tsp	minced gingerroot	2 mL

1. In a saucepan, combine papaya, water, coconut milk and ginger. Bring to a boil over medium heat. Reduce heat to low and simmer until papaya is soft, 5 to 7 minutes.

2. Transfer to a blender or use an immersion blender in the saucepan. Purée until smooth. Let cool until warm to the touch or transfer to an airtight container and refrigerate for up to 3 days.

Nutrients per serving (½ cup/125 mL)	
Calories 80	Dietary fiber . . . . . . 1.6 g
Protein . . . . 0.9 g	Sodium . . . . 7.0 mg
Total fat . . . . 6.1 g	Calcium . . . . 19.0 mg
Saturated fat. . . . . . 5.4 g	Iron . . . . 0.5 mg
Carbohydrates. . . . . 6.9 g	Vitamin C. . . . . . 35.3 mg

Not just for babies
This is a wonderful dip for Mom and Dad with grilled shrimp and a garnish of toasted shredded coconut. The flavors will transport you to Hawaii.

Oven-Roasted Artichokes

In my opinion, this is the way artichokes were meant to be eaten!

Makes about 2 cups (500 mL)

■ ■ ■

Chef Jordan's Tips

If turkey bacon doesn't appeal to you, a nitrate-free smoked turkey breast or thigh works just as well. Break up the turkey into small pieces and follow the recipe as written.

Artichokes are flower buds that are eaten prior to budding. The artichoke can range in color from light green to dark purple/red and in size from the baby, which can be 3 inches (7.5 cm) long to the Lyon, which can grow to 6 to 7 inches (15 to 17.5 cm) in length. Although a tremendous amount of work, baby artichokes are one of my favorite garnishes for meat or poultry dishes.

- Preheat oven to 400°F (200°C)
- Ovenproof skillet

2	fresh artichokes (about 1½ lbs/750 g)	2
1 tbsp	extra virgin olive oil	15 mL
¼ cup	finely diced nitrate-free turkey bacon	50 mL
¼ cup	finely diced sweet onion	50 mL
2	cloves garlic, minced	2
1	sprig fresh thyme	1
¼ cup	freshly grated Parmesan cheese	50 mL
2 tbsp	water	25 mL

1. Remove artichoke stems and set aside. Trim off the top two-thirds of each artichoke and remove the bright green leaves, exposing the whitish leaves. Plunge a spoon into the middle of the choke, removing the thorny middle leaves and exposing the heart. Cut artichokes into 4 slices.

2. Peel the outer portion of the stems, leaving the tender white core in the middle. Slice the stems.

3. In an ovenproof skillet, heat oil over medium heat. Add bacon, onion, garlic and thyme and sauté until onion is soft, 3 to 4 minutes.

4. Stir in artichokes and stems and transfer skillet to preheated oven. Roast, stirring often to prevent bacon from burning, until artichokes are fork tender, about 25 minutes. Remove from oven and stir in Parmesan cheese and water. Cut to desired size. Let cool until warm to the touch or transfer to an airtight container and refrigerate for up to 3 days.

Nutrients per serving (½ cup/125 mL)	
Calories 156	Dietary fiber ..... 10.2 g
Protein .... 9.8 g	Sodium ...... 399.3 mg
Total fat .... 6.0 g	Calcium .... 53.0 mg
Saturated fat...... 1.6 g	Iron .... 0.2 mg
Carbohydrates.... 21.7 g	Vitamin C....... 1.3 mg

Not just for babies

Where was this recipe when my wife, Tamar, introduced me to artichokes years ago? Artichokes were a staple in my wife's family, but they boiled them and served them with mayonnaise, which wasn't particularly appetizing. Perhaps many people haven't attempted to roast artichokes before. I encourage you to give it a try. I think you'll enjoy them.

Nutrition Tip

Artichokes are a nutrient-dense food, packed with fiber, minerals, vitamin C and folate. They also contain a powerful antioxidant called cynarin, which protects the liver from chemical and environmental toxins and helps it to regenerate healthy tissue.

Quick Mushroom Soup

This recipe epitomizes what I call "simple elegance" — basic in method and refined in taste.

**Makes about
5 cups (1.25 L)**

▪ ▪ ▪

Chef Jordan's Tips

Jonah loved this
mushroom soup from
the get-go but it's taken
him almost four years
to fully appreciate
mushrooms and their
many varieties. Oyster,
shiitake and portobello
are now some of his
favorites.

Nutrition Tip

Mushrooms are a
delicious way to ensure
there is enough folate
in your baby's diet.
All types of mushrooms
contain folate, a
B vitamin that is
important for your
baby's healthy growth
and development.
Among other functions,
folate is essential for the
formation of red and
white blood cells in the
bone marrow.

1 tbsp	unsalted butter	15 mL
5 cups	sliced mushrooms	1.25 L
1 cup	diced white onions	250 mL
¾ cup	finely diced peeled carrots	175 mL
3	cloves garlic, minced	3
2	fresh sage leaves	2
3 cups	Roasted Chicken Stock (see recipe, page 202)	750 mL
1 cup	whole milk	250 mL
1 tsp	extra virgin olive oil	5 mL

1. In a large pot, melt butter over high heat. Add mushrooms, onions, carrots, garlic and sage and sauté until carrots are soft, about 10 minutes. Add chicken stock and milk and bring to a boil. Reduce heat to low and simmer until carrots are falling apart, about 30 minutes.

2. Add olive oil. Transfer to a blender or use an immersion blender in the pot. Purée until smooth. Let cool until warm to the touch or transfer to an airtight container and refrigerate for up to 3 days.

Nutrients per serving (½ cup/125 mL)	
Calories 128	Dietary fiber . . . . . . 1.7 g
Protein . . . . 7.9 g	Sodium . . . . 50.6 mg
Total fat . . . . 7.6 g	Calcium . . . . 53.1 mg
Saturated fat. . . . . . 2.7 g	Iron . . . . 0.8 mg
Carbohydrates. . . . . 7.8 g	Vitamin C. . . . . . . 5.9 mg

Not just for babies
This is a delicious soup everyone in the family can enjoy together. Mom and Dad, bon appetit.

Corn and Chickpea Chowder

Although it's a bit of extra work to roast the corn for this chowder, it creates a distinctly "out of the ordinary" flavor. It's definitely worth the effort.

Makes about 4½ cups (1.125 L)

■ ■ ■

Chef Jordan's Tips

To roast corn, place 4 ears on a preheated barbecue (500°F/260°C). Cook, rotating often, until the husk is dark brown, about 20 minutes. (The corn will not be fully cooked.) Let cool for at least 5 minutes. Remove husks and silks by hand and, using a sharp knife and working over a container, trim away the kernels. Scrape the cob, which releases all of the milky juices that develop the flavor in your chowder.

Nutrition Tip

When putting together a meal for your toddler, it is important to make sure it is balanced. The chickpeas in this chowder provide protein for building muscle and the corn provides carbohydrates to fuel physical activity. To round out the meal, add a green vegetable such as Sautéed Swiss Chard.

1 tbsp	unsalted butter	15 mL
1½ cups	roasted fresh corn kernels	375 mL
1½ cups	cooked chickpeas, drained and rinsed (see page 77)	375 mL
1	roasted red bell pepper, peeled, seeded and diced	1
1 tbsp	diced lean nitrate-free bacon, optional (see Tips, page 93)	15 mL
1 tbsp	minced garlic	15 mL
3¼ cups	water or stock	700 mL

1. In a saucepan, melt butter over medium heat. Add corn, chickpeas, red pepper, bacon and garlic and cook, stirring, for 5 minutes. Add water and bring to a boil. Reduce heat to low and simmer until chickpeas are very soft, about 35 minutes.

2. Transfer to a blender or use an immersion blender in the saucepan. Pulse to desired consistency. Let cool until warm to the touch or transfer to an airtight container and refrigerate for up to 3 days or freeze for up to 3 months.

Nutrients per serving (½ cup/125 mL)	
Calories 55	Dietary fiber . . . . . . 1.7 g
Protein . . . . 1.9 g	Sodium . . . . 7.9 mg
Total fat . . . . 1.9 g	Calcium . . . . 10.4 mg
Saturated fat . . . . . . 0.9 g	Iron . . . . 0.5 mg
Carbohydrates . . . . . 8.8 g	Vitamin C . . . . . . 19.2 mg

Not just for babies
Add 1 cup (250 mL) shredded roasted duck meat after serving your baby.

Asparagus and Roasted Tomato

This flavor combination, asparagus and roasted tomato, is one that adults really enjoy. Your baby will love it, too.

**Makes about
2 cups (500 mL)**

Chef Jordan's Tips

Peel your asparagus for the best result. As tender as asparagus can be, it may still be fibrous, making it tough for children to chew. To peel asparagus, use a vegetable peeler. Peel from under the tip all the way down the stalk, rotating until all of the whitish flesh is exposed. I guarantee you'll be peeling your asparagus from this point forward.

Nutrition Tip

When we think of potassium, we often think of bananas, but tomatoes are also a significant source of this important mineral. Potassium is one of the body's main electrolytes, which means it generates electrical impulses that keep your nervous system working. This function can become unbalanced when your baby suffers from vomiting or diarrhea.

- Preheat oven to 350°F (180°C)
- Rimmed baking sheet

½ cup	cherry tomatoes	125 mL
8 oz	asparagus, trimmed and cut in half	250 g
2 cups	water or Roasted Chicken Stock (see recipe, page 202) or Vegetable Stock (see recipe, page 201)	500 mL
2	basil leaves	2

1. On baking sheet, roast tomatoes in preheated oven until soft and skins begin to split, about 20 minutes. Transfer to a saucepan and add asparagus and water. Bring to a boil over medium heat. Reduce heat to low and simmer until asparagus is tender and liquid has reduced by one-quarter, about 8 minutes.

2. Add basil leaves. Transfer to a blender or use an immersion blender in the saucepan. Pulse to desired consistency. Let cool until warm to the touch or transfer to an airtight container and refrigerate for up to 3 days.

Nutrients per serving (½ cup/125 mL)	
Calories 23	Dietary fiber . . . . . . 1.7 g
Protein . . . . 1.6 g	Sodium . . . . 5.3 mg
Total fat . . . . 0.1 g	Calcium . . . . 20.7 mg
Saturated fat. . . . . . 0.0 g	Iron . . . . 0.3 mg
Carbohydrates. . . . . 3.9 g	Vitamin C. . . . . . 10.1 mg

Not just for babies

Try serving this as a cold soup with grated old Cheddar cheese. Add about ½ cup (125 mL) stock to 1 cup (250 mL) of the purée.

The Vegetarian Baby

Celebrate Spring

For a farmer, spring means the ground has thawed and is soft enough to plant. For a gardener it's the first lovely blooms on previously bare trees. For me, it means the arrival of certain foods such as the first locally grown asparagus, which is my favorite springtime delicacy. I love the tender stalks and sweet flavor of this beautiful vegetable. Used in combination with tomato and basil, as it is in the recipe opposite, asparagus creates a fabulous contrast in textures. Asparagus is as versatile a food as they come. It can be served on its own, as a simple side or in salads, and combines beautifully with many other ingredients — not only those featured opposite but also those in my recipe for Alaskan Halibut en Papillote (see recipe, page 152).

A vegetarian or vegan diet can be a healthy choice for your baby, so long as it is well planned. The more restricted it is, the more carefully you'll need to plan to ensure your baby gets the full range of nutrients she needs to grow and develop properly. Because many of the nutrients your baby needs are easier to get from animal products — for instance, protein, iron, vitamin B_{12} and vitamin D, you will want to pay particular attention to ensuring that her diet includes foods that are rich in these nutrients.

For the first year or so of your baby's life, breast milk and formula will provide vitamin B_{12}. If the nursing mother is a strict vegetarian or vegan, she will need to make sure she is getting enough supplemental B_{12} to ensure there is enough in her breast milk. Subsequently, the baby may be able to obtain an adequate supply of this nutrient from milk and dairy products. After weaning, vegans may need to specifically look for foods fortified with this crucial vitamin, such as fortified soy products and fortified plant milks such as rice or almond milk.

Good sources of protein are eggs, yogurt, cheese, soy products, such as tofu, and beans and lentils. After your baby passes her first birthday (depending on the family history of allergies) nuts and seeds can also be added to her diet to provide protein.

Iron is found in whole grains such as millet and quinoa, dark green vegetables, such as broccoli and spinach, lentils, beans and soy products, and dried apricots.

Vitamin D is found mostly in fortified milk and fatty fish such as salmon, mackerel and sardines, but the best source is unprotected (meaning no sunscreen), but safe exposure to the sun. Consult your pediatrician for the appropriate guidelines.

Fennel and Orange Sauté

In this recipe, the sweet and sour flavor of the oranges complements the fennel beautifully, toning down its licorice flavor. Your baby will love the very mild licorice flavor of the fennel.

Makes about ¾ cup (175 mL)

■ ■ ■

Chef Jordan's Tips
When available, clementines add a unique flavor that is slightly different from oranges but would be awesome in this recipe!

Nutrition Tip
Because you are using the peel, we strongly recommend the use of organic oranges in this recipe. The chemical residue of dyes, waxes and pesticides is concentrated in the skin of most conventionally grown fruit. Every day your baby is exposed to environmental and chemical toxins and this is one small step you can take to limit this exposure.

* Potato masher, optional

1 tsp	unsalted butter	5 mL
1¾ cups	finely diced fresh fennel	425 mL
1 tbsp	grated orange zest	15 mL
⅓ cup	freshly squeezed orange juice	75 mL

1. In a saucepan, melt butter over medium heat. Add fennel and sauté until soft, about 10 minutes. Stir in orange zest and juice. Reduce heat to low and simmer until liquid has evaporated, about 5 minutes. Mash or cut to desired consistency. Let cool until warm to the touch or transfer to an airtight container and refrigerate for up to 3 days.

Nutrients per serving (½ cup/125 mL)	
Calories 82	Dietary fiber . . . . . . 3.7 g
Protein . . . . 1.7 g	Sodium . . . . 53.8 mg
Total fat . . . . 2.8 g	Calcium . . . . 61.8 mg
Saturated fat. . . . . . 1.6 g	Iron . . . . 0.8 mg
Carbohydrates. . . . 14.1 g	Vitamin C . . . . . . 38.2 mg

Not just for babies
Your baby will love this on its own, but Mom and Dad will probably prefer it as a condiment. My family uses this as a relish for hamburgers and hot dogs or even on a ham sandwich.

"Smashed" Baby Potatoes

I recently made this for my son and his response was, "They tastes like French fries, Daddy." And no frying necessary.

Makes 8 to 10 servings

■ ■ ■

Chef Jordan's Tips

Leftover smashed potatoes can be used to make an excellent cold potato salad. Freshly squeezed lemon juice, fresh chives and mayonnaise complete a very tasty "leftover."

Nutrition Tip

It is important to consider the type of oil you use when cooking at high temperatures, because when oils are overheated, free radicals and other unhealthy products form. Butter and olive and coconut oils, to name a few, have a sturdy structure and do not change substantially when heated to below their smoking point. Seed or nut oils such as flax, pumpkin or walnut are extremely sensitive to heat and easily oxidize when heated. Oxidized fats represent considerable health risks in cardiovascular disease.

2 lbs	small new potatoes	1 kg
12 cups	water	3 L
2 tbsp	extra virgin olive oil	25 mL

1. In a large pot, combine potatoes and water. Bring to a boil over medium heat. Reduce heat and simmer until fork tender, about 20 minutes. Drain and transfer potatoes to a baking sheet.

2. Preheat oven to 350°F (180°C).

3. Using the bottom of a second baking sheet, cover the potatoes and press down to crush, essentially flattening them into a thick chunky pancake. Drizzle half the olive oil on the potatoes, turn and drizzle with remainder.

4. Roast in preheated oven until crispy, about 20 minutes. Transfer to a plate and let cool until warm to the touch or transfer to an airtight container and refrigerate for up to 3 days.

Nutrients per serving	
Calories 106	Dietary fiber . . . . . . 1.9 g
Protein . . . . 2.1 g	Sodium . . . . 18.1 mg
Total fat . . . . 3.1 g	Calcium . . . . 22.6 mg
Saturated fat. . . . . . 0.5 g	Iron . . . . 0.8 mg
Carbohydrates. . . . 18.0 g	Vitamin C. . . . . . . 9.8 mg

Not just for babies

This is one dish you'll enjoy every bit as much as your baby. Bon appetit.

Crispy Potato Galette

Potato galette makes an excellent snack in place of store-bought potato chips, and it's much tastier, too.

Makes about 4 servings

∎ ∎ ∎

Chef Jordan's Tips

Believe it or not, this galette stores well in the refrigerator. To reheat, bake in a preheated (350°F/180°C) oven until crisp, about 5 minutes.

Nutrition Tip

Scrub your potatoes well and keep the skins on. That's where all the nutrients are concentrated, especially potassium, which every cell of your baby's body requires. Don't use potatoes that are the least bit green or have any sprouts. Both indicate the presence of solanine, which can detrimentally affect collagen repair, important for your baby's bones and joints.

| 2 tbsp | extra virgin olive oil | 25 mL |
| 1 cup | grated baking potato, skin on | 250 mL |

1. In a small nonstick skillet, heat olive oil over high heat. Add potato, covering the entire surface of the pan and evenly distributing to create what looks like a small pizza crust. Reduce heat to low and cook until bottom is golden brown, about 10 minutes. Flip and cook until second side is golden brown and potatoes are tender, about 10 minutes.

2. Transfer to a plate and let cool until warm to the touch or wrap in plastic wrap and refrigerate for up to 3 days. To serve, cut into wedges.

Nutrients per serving	
Calories 141	Dietary fiber . . . . . . 2.5 g
Protein . . . . 2.3 g	Sodium . . . . 6.8 mg
Total fat . . . . 6.0 g	Calcium . . . . 13.6 mg
Saturated fat . . . . . . 0.9 g	Iron . . . . 0.9 mg
Carbohydrates . . . . 19.8 g	Vitamin C . . . . . . 22.3 mg

Not just for babies

One of my signature dishes and a personal favorite is a Baby Spinach Salad with Smoked Salmon and Potato Galette. After warming the galette, layer 3 large slices (about 2 oz/60 g) of smoked salmon and squeeze about 1 tsp (5 mL) fresh lemon juice over top. Toss about 1½ cups (375 mL) of baby spinach in 1 tsp (5 mL) extra virgin olive oil and a drizzle of champagne or cider vinegar. Season with a pinch of kosher salt and freshly ground black pepper. Place the salad over top of the galette and serve.

Broccoli, Potato and Spinach Pie

This "crustless" pie is a huge hit in my family; I am sure it will be in yours as well.

Makes about 8 servings

∎ ∎ ∎

Chef Jordan's Tips

If you prefer, substitute ½ cup (125 mL) whole milk for the heavy cream in this recipe.

If you have the opportunity to buy sorrel, which is available at farmers' markets throughout the summer, substitute an equal quantity for the spinach. It has bright green leaves with jagged edges and a bitter citrus flavor that complements the flavors beautifully.

Nutrition Tip

Spinach is second only to kale as the highest vegetable source of the mineral calcium. It also contains a significant amount of iron.

Buy organic potatoes and spinach

- Preheat oven to 300°F (150°C)
- 9-inch (23 cm) pie plate

1 lb	red new potatoes (about 4 small), thinly sliced	500 g
2 tsp	melted unsalted butter	10 mL
4 cups	baby spinach	1 L
1 cup	chopped broccoli florets	250 mL
¾ cup	whipping (35%) cream	175 mL
¾ cup	freshly grated Parmesan cheese	175 mL

1. In a mixing bowl, combine potatoes and butter, tossing until well coated. Transfer to pie plate, overlapping as necessary. Bake in preheated oven until potatoes are soft, about 25 minutes.

2. In a bowl combine spinach, broccoli, cream and cheese. Pour over potatoes and bake until liquid is thick and potatoes are fork tender, about 20 minutes. Mash or cut to desired consistency. Let cool until warm to the touch or wrap in plastic wrap and refrigerate for up to 3 days.

Nutrients per serving	
Calories 185	Dietary fiber . . . . . . 1.6 g
Protein . . . . 5.0 g	Sodium . . . . . . 149.5 mg
Total fat . . . . 12.8 g	Calcium . . . . . . 111.9 mg
Saturated fat. . . . . . 7.9 g	Iron . . . . 0.9 mg
Carbohydrates. . . . 13.1 g	Vitamin C. . . . . . . 9.0 mg

Not just for babies
Garnish the pie with soft goat cheese and thin strands of fresh basil...bon appetit!

Grilled Asparagus with Three Cheeses

I love how the cheese melts together to cover the asparagus, and Jonah loves that he can eat the spears with his hands. Who am I kidding? I like eating with my hands, too.

Makes about 2½ cups (625 mL) diced

■ ■ ■

Chef Jordan's Tips

So many of my friends cook their asparagus directly on the barbecue without "blanching" (boiling) it first. Mine are a beautifully green and crunchy and theirs are grey black and quite "woody." There is really no comparison.

Nutrition Tip

Asparagus contains inulin, a carbohydrate that helps to promote the growth of friendly bacteria in your baby's gut. Inulin is resistant to digestion in the small intestine so it reaches the large intestine, or colon, largely intact. Here it is fermented by and provides fuel for the friendly healthy intestinal bacteria that are a key component of your baby's immune system. Garlic and leeks are other good sources of inulin.

- Preheat barbecue to high (500°F/260°C)
- Potato masher, optional

8 cups	water	2 L
1 lb	asparagus, peeled (see Tips, page 128)	500 g
¼ cup	freshly grated Parmesan cheese	50 mL
¼ cup	shredded Cheddar cheese	50 mL
1 tbsp	finely diced Brie cheese	15 mL

1. In a saucepan, bring water to a rolling boil over medium heat. Add asparagus and cook until vibrant green and soft, about 3 minutes. Drain well. Place asparagus on the preheated grill until grill marks appear, about 2 minutes.

2. In a bowl, combine asparagus, Parmesan, Cheddar and Brie cheeses. Mash or cut to desired consistency. Let cool until warm to the touch or transfer to an airtight container and refrigerate for up to 3 days.

Nutrients per serving (½ cup/125 mL)	
Calories 70	Dietary fiber . . . . . . 2.0 g
Protein . . . . 5.0 g	Sodium . . . . . . 122.7 mg
Total fat . . . . 3.5 g	Calcium . . . . . . 123.6 mg
Saturated fat. . . . . . 2.2 g	Iron . . . . 0.4 mg
Carbohydrates. . . . . 4.3 g	Vitamin C. . . . . . . 8.8 mg

Not Just for babies

My sister Jennifer, the sort-of vegetarian of the family, requests this dish every Friday evening in the summer months. If she didn't I would probably still make it — I love it, too.

Red Potato Salad with Cheddar Cheese and Boiled Eggs

Most of the potato salads I remember from my childhood would cause me to run an extra 30 minutes on the treadmill to work off the calories. They were full of mayonnaise or oil or both, in the case of my late Gramma Jean's. In this recipe, the combination of chopped boiled egg with grated carrots creates a wonderful texture I'm sure your baby will enjoy.

Makes about 2 cups (500 mL)

■ ■ ■

Chef Jordan's Tips
A unique addition to this recipe would be whole quail eggs. Now readily available in specialty shops, quail eggs contribute sophistication without adding effort. About $\frac{1}{5}$ the size of chicken eggs, they can be served whole.

Nutrition Tip
Which came first, the chicken or the egg? In this case it's the feed the chicken eats. You can increase your baby's consumption of omega-3 fats by buying eggs that are richer in this nutrient. When chickens are fed flax seeds their eggs contain more of these beneficial fats. Look for them in the supermarket.

1¾ cups	cubed red potatoes	425 mL
2	hard-cooked eggs, chopped	2
½ cup	grated peeled carrots	125 mL
⅓ cup	shredded Cheddar cheese	75 mL

1. In a saucepan, cover potatoes with cold water. Bring to a boil over medium heat. Reduce heat to low and simmer until fork tender, about 20 minutes. Drain well. Let cool to room temperature.

2. In a bowl, combine eggs, carrots and cheese. Stir in potatoes. Cover and refrigerate overnight or for up to 3 days.

Nutrients per serving (½ cup/125 mL)

Calories	137	Dietary fiber	1.3 g
Protein	6.7 g	Sodium	105.3 mg
Total fat	5.2 g	Calcium	83.1 mg
Saturated fat	2.7 g	Iron	1.1 mg
Carbohydrates	15.4 g	Vitamin C	17.0 mg

Not just for babies
Mom and Dad, after scooping off some for your baby, add 1 tbsp (15 mL) red wine vinegar and a pinch each of kosher salt and freshly ground pepper.

Best-Ever Barbecued Corn

I love compound butters. This chive version is particularly delicious with corn.

Makes about 12 servings

Chef Jordan's Tips

A great version of this recipe: Before grilling, peel a portion of the husk back but do not remove it. Rub the exposed corn with unsalted butter. Repeat until the entire cob has been buttered, replacing all the husks and pulling them together.

Nutrition Tip

We think butter is better than margarine. It is high in vitamins A, E and D and the antioxidant selenium. Butter contains butyric acid and lauric acid, both of which contribute to a healthy immune system. It also contains cholesterol, which is present in large amounts in breast milk. Cholesterol is crucial for your baby's brain and nervous system development and is a precursor to the important fat-soluble vitamin D, which is needed for proper growth, healthy bones and strong immune function.

• Preheat barbecue to medium-high (400°F/200°C)

6	ears corn, husks on (see Tips, left)	6
2 tbsp	unsalted butter, at room temperature	25 mL
1 tbsp	finely chopped chives	15 mL

1. Place corn on preheated barbecue. Cover and cook, rotating the corn often, until the husk is dark brown all over, about 20 minutes. Transfer to a plate and let cool for at least 5 minutes before you attempt to husk the corn. Remove husks and silks. Cut the corn cobs into thirds.

2. In a bowl, combine butter and chives. Add the corn and toss to thoroughly coat. Let cool until warm to the touch or transfer to an airtight container and refrigerate for up to 3 days.

Nutrients per serving			
Calories	89	Dietary fiber	3.5 g
Protein	2.5 g	Sodium	5.2 mg
Total fat	3.1 g	Calcium	30.7 mg
Saturated fat	1.5 g	Iron	0.5 mg
Carbohydrates	13.0 g	Vitamin C	3.5 mg

Not just for babies

Compound butters (softened butter combined with other flavors, such as fresh herbs) are delicious on everything from pasta to fish and pancakes to eggs. The method is simple. Incorporate any seasoning into room temperature butter, roll the butter in parchment paper, label (so you don't forget what's inside) and freeze for up to 6 months. As needed, remove the roll of butter and cut a piece off, returning the butter to the freezer for later use.

Oven-Roasted Cauliflower with Fresh Herbs

About five years ago, I showed my mother this recipe and it's become one of her favorites. Since then, it has graced her table at most family meals. Please, Mom, we love oven-roasted cauliflower, but not ALL the time!

Makes about 5 cups (1.25 L)

Chef Jordan's Tips

Fresh goat cheese is a nice addition to this recipe. In a bowl, toss the cauliflower, right from the oven, with ¼ cup (50 mL) soft goat cheese.

Nutrition Tip

When cruciferous vegetables such as cauliflower, broccoli, cabbage and Brussels sprouts are chopped or chewed, a compound called sulforaphane is formed. Research shows that this compound triggers the liver to produce enzymes that detoxify cancer-causing chemicals. Human population studies show that diets high in cruciferous vegetables are associated with reduced incidence of certain cancers. It is never too early to establish healthy eating habits.

- Preheat oven to 350°F (180°C)
- Rimmed baking sheet

2	heads cauliflower, cut into florets (about 4 lbs/2 kg)	2
¼ cup	extra virgin olive oil	50 mL
2 tbsp	chopped fresh parsley	25 mL
1 tbsp	chopped fresh thyme	15 mL

1. In a bowl, combine cauliflower and oil, mixing thoroughly to evenly coat. Spread evenly on baking sheet and roast in preheated oven until golden brown, about 30 minutes.

2. Add parsley and thyme and toss to coat. Let cool until warm to the touch or transfer to an airtight container and refrigerate for up to 3 days.

Nutrients per serving (½ cup/125 mL)	
Calories 89	Dietary fiber . . . . . . 4.6 g
Protein . . . . 3.6 g	Sodium . . . . 54.9 mg
Total fat . . . . 4.9 g	Calcium . . . . 41.9 mg
Saturated fat. . . . . . 0.7 g	Iron . . . . 0.9 mg
Carbohydrates. . . . . 9.7 g	Vitamin C. . . . . . 85.6 mg

Not just for babies

To create a dish that is "over the top," separate off a portion for Baby and season the remainder with a pinch of kosher salt and freshly ground black pepper before roasting. It doesn't need anything else.

Jonah's "Mac and Cheese"

This is the only version of macaroni and cheese my son, Jonah, has known for the first four years of his life, and he can't get enough of it. I recommend making extras for you, Mom and Dad!

Makes about
2¼ cups (550 mL)

■ ■ ■

Chef Jordan's Tips

Feel free to use your noodle of choice, from shorter noodles like penne to the longer linguine. For added nutrition choose whole-grain versions, such as those made from whole wheat, spelt, Kamut or farro.

Nutrition Tip

All pasta, white or not, is moderate on the glycemic index. This index is the measurement of the rate at which carbohydrates are digested and converted into glucose (your body's energy source). Moderate and low glycemic foods help balance blood sugar and provide a prolonged release of energy. Whole-grain pastas have the same glycemic values but contain a full range of nutrients, unlike their processed counterparts, and are much higher in fiber.

5 cups	water	1.25 L
1 cup	farfellini (small bow ties) pasta	250 mL
½ cup	Roasted Sweet Potato Purée (see recipe, page 42)	125 mL
¼ cup	freshly grated Parmesan cheese	50 mL
2 tbsp	sour cream	25 mL

1. In a large pot, bring water to a boil over high heat. Add pasta and cook, stirring often, until soft, about 20 minutes. Reserving 1 cup (250 mL) of the cooking water, drain pasta.

2. Return pasta and reserved water to the pot over low heat. Stir in sweet potato purée, Parmesan cheese and sour cream. Cook, stirring, until mixture is thick and noodles are evenly coated, 2 to 3 minutes. Cut to desired consistency. Let cool until warm to the touch or transfer to an airtight container and refrigerate for up to 3 days.

Nutrients per serving (½ cup/125 mL)	
Calories 100	Dietary fiber . . . . . . 1.1 g
Protein . . . . 4.1 g	Sodium . . . . 88.8 mg
Total fat . . . . 2.7 g	Calcium . . . . 69.8 mg
Saturated fat. . . . . . 1.6 g	Iron . . . . 0.6 mg
Carbohydrates. . . . 14.2 g	Vitamin C. . . . . . . 0.4 mg

Not Just for babies

The addition of freshly ground allspice and chopped fresh oregano transforms this rustic dish into a sophisticated meal.

Basic Pearled Barley

Barley has become a staple in my home. The texture is so versatile that it easily substitutes for rice or pasta.

Makes about 5 cups (1.25 L)

■ ■ ■

Chef Jordan's Tips

Toasting really enhances the flavor of barley.

Pearled and pot barley are found in the dry sections of supermarkets next to the rice and beans. To purchase whole (hulled) barley, you'll usually have to visit a natural foods store. If desired, substitute pot or whole barley for the pearled version in this recipe. Cover the pot after bringing to a boil and increase the cooking time to about 45 minutes for pot barley and 1 hour or more for the whole-grain version.

Nutrition Tip

Pearled barley cooks reasonably quickly and has a nice texture and taste. However, since most of the bran and germ have been removed, it does not have the full range of nutrients that the whole-grain version provides.

2 cups	pearled barley	500 mL
1 tbsp	unsalted butter	15 mL
5½ cups	water, Vegetable Stock (see recipe, page 201) or Roasted Chicken Stock (see recipe, page 202)	1.375 mL

1. In a sieve, rinse barley thoroughly under cold, running water removing possible impurities, until water runs clear, about 1 minute. Drain well.

2. In a saucepan, melt butter over medium heat. Add barley and toast, stirring constantly, until golden brown, about 5 minutes.

3. Add water and bring to a boil. Reduce heat to low and simmer until most of the liquid has been absorbed, about 30 minutes. Let cool until warm to the touch or transfer to an airtight container and refrigerate for up to 3 days.

Nutrients per serving (½ cup/125 mL)	
Calories 154	Dietary fiber . . . . . . 6.4 g
Protein . . . . 4.0 g	Sodium . . . . 7.3 mg
Total fat . . . . 2.0 g	Calcium . . . . 12.2 mg
Saturated fat. . . . . . 0.7 g	Iron . . . . 0.9 mg
Carbohydrates. . . . 31.2 g	Vitamin C. . . . . . . 0.0 mg

Not Just for babies

Barley is so versatile it can be served as the feature ingredient in salads, both hot and cold, under stews or as an accompaniment to stir-fries instead of rice. I've made a big batch here so you can make it part of your meal after serving some to your baby. It also stores well.

Warm Barley with Fresh Herbs and Parmesan Cheese

If your children love the taste of macaroni and cheese, just wait until they try this "gourmet" version.

Makes about 1½ cups (375 mL)

■ ■ ■

Chef Jordan's Tips

I use fresh herbs a lot because they impart a unique freshness and flavor to dishes. When you introduce this recipe to your baby, start with equal parts of flat-leaf parsley and basil, which will produce a mildly flavored result. After a while, add some stronger tasting herbs, such as tarragon or oregano.

Nutrition Tip

Because of its digestibility, doctors in Italy recommend Parmesan cheese for babies. Its long aging process essentially predigests the proteins in milk, making them readily available for the body to use. Parmesan cheese does not have any lactose, which makes it a great choice if you suspect your baby can't tolerate dairy or is allergic to it.

1½ cups	cooked barley (see recipe, page 139)	375 mL
1 tbsp	unsalted butter	15 mL
⅓ cup	freshly grated Parmesan cheese	75 mL
¼ cup	chopped fresh herbs (see Tips, left)	50 mL

1. In a saucepan, melt butter over medium heat. Add barley and cook, stirring, until warm, about 3 minutes. Stir in Parmesan cheese and herbs. Let cool until warm to the touch or transfer to an airtight container and refrigerate for up to 3 days.

Nutrients per serving (½ cup/125 mL)	
Calories 168	Dietary fiber . . . . . . 3.1 g
Protein . . . . 5.2 g	Sodium . . . . . . 133.4 mg
Total fat . . . . 6.6 g	Calcium . . . . . . 108.7 mg
Saturated fat. . . . . . 4.0 g	Iron . . . . 1.3 mg
Carbohydrates. . . . 22.7 g	Vitamin C. . . . . . . 3.1 mg

Not just for babies

In a saucepan, over medium heat, cook ¼ cup (50 mL) white wine and 1 tsp (5 mL) butter until reduced by half. Scoop off about 1¼ cups (300 mL) of the warm barley mixture and combine with the wine reduction. This makes an awesome side dish.

Millet and Cauliflower with Fresh Oregano

If you and your child are not accustomed to eating millet, here's a great recipe. The familiar undertones in the cauliflower and oregano will help you to adjust to the new taste.

Makes about 3 cups (750 mL)

Chef Jordan's Tips

After the millet is cooked, I prefer to use a potato masher rather than puréeing to achieve the desired texture. It resembles mashed potatoes — nice and fluffy.

Nutrition Tip

Oregano, like many herbs, is known for its medicinal properties. Fresh oregano actually contains 42 times as much antioxidant activity as apples. In fact, it has more of this cell-protecting quality than any other herb.

- Potato masher

½ cup	millet	125 mL
2½ cups	water or Vegetable Stock (see recipe, page 201) or Roasted Chicken Stock (see recipe, page 202)	625 mL
2¼ cups	chopped cauliflower florets	550 mL
1 tsp	chopped fresh oregano	5 mL

1. In a saucepan, toast millet over medium heat, stirring, until golden brown, 2 to 3 minutes.

2. Add water and cauliflower and bring to a boil. Reduce heat to low and simmer until all water has evaporated, about 25 minutes.

3. Transfer to a bowl and add oregano. Using a potato masher, mash until smooth. Let cool until warm to the touch or transfer to an airtight container and refrigerate for up to 3 days.

Nutrients per serving (½ cup/125 mL)	
Calories 73	Dietary fiber . . . . . . 2.4 g
Protein . . . . 2.6 g	Sodium . . . . 15.6 mg
Total fat . . . . 0.8 g	Calcium . . . . 14.0 mg
Saturated fat. . . . . . 0.1 g	Iron . . . . 0.7 mg
Carbohydrates. . . . 14.2 g	Vitamin C. . . . . . 18.1 mg

Not just for babies

Set aside 1 cup (250 mL) of the mixture. Add ½ cup (125 mL) each roasted corn kernels and chopped tomato, 1 tbsp (15 mL) freshly squeezed lemon juice and salt and pepper, to taste.

Creamy Brown Rice and Fresh Basil

This savory rice pudding will be a great hit with your children! The creamy texture mimics a traditional dessert rice pudding, but it is infused with the flavor of basil.

Makes about 1¼ cups (300 mL)

■ ■ ■

Chef Jordan's Tips
Virtually any rice will work in place of brown rice. From sushi rice to jasmine rice — they all make great rice pudding. Just be sure to adjust your cooking time to suit the grain of choice. Faster cooking rice, such as jasmine, may take only about 1¼ hours.

Nutrition Tip
Unlike white rice, brown rice has only had its outer hull removed so it retains much of its original nutritional value. It is also very high in the mineral manganese, which is important for producing energy in your baby's body. Brown rice has about four times as much fiber as white rice and does not contain gluten so is safe for those who have problems digesting gluten.

4 cups	whole milk	1 L
½ cup	long-grain brown rice	125 mL
2	basil leaves	2

1. In a saucepan, combine milk, rice and basil. Bring to a boil over medium heat. Reduce heat to low and simmer, stirring occasionally, until most of the milk has been absorbed and the rice becomes soft, about 2 hours. Let cool until warm to the touch or transfer to an airtight container and refrigerate for up to 2 days.

Nutrients per serving (½ cup/125 mL)	
Calories 278	Dietary fiber . . . . . . 0.7 g
Protein . . . . 13.5 g	Sodium . . . . . . 156.6 mg
Total fat . . . . 13.0 g	Calcium . . . . . . 445.7 mg
Saturated fat. . . . . . 7.4 g	Iron . . . . 0.3 mg
Carbohydrates. . . . 26.8 g	Vitamin C. . . . . . . 0.1 mg

Not just for babies
There's no rule that states rice pudding is only for dessert. Preheat your oven to 350°F (180°C). On a baking sheet drizzle 1 tbsp (15 mL) extra virgin olive oil. Add 2 minced cloves of garlic with 2 cups (500 mL) of your favorite mushrooms cut into bite-size pieces (button, portobello, shiitake, chanterelle would all work) and toss well. Roast until soft, about 20 minutes. Place on top of ¾ cup (175 mL) of the rice pudding. Garnish with 2 tbsp (25 mL) creamy goat cheese.

Soft Polenta with Cheddar Cheese and Broccoli Florets

Your children will come to love this flavor combination of cornmeal, broccoli and cheese.

Makes about 3½ cups (875 mL)

■ ■ ■

Chef Jordan's Tips

I use the term "bloom" to describe the process in which the cornmeal opens up and absorbs the water, literally expanding.

If you are using stone-ground cornmeal, increase the quantity of water to 4½ cups (1.125 L).

Nutrition Tip

Extra-old cheddar cheese is a good source of calcium, which you know your baby needs for growing teeth. Even better is the fact that the extra-old cheese increases saliva flow, which washes away acids and sugars that contribute to tooth decay. It is never too soon to get a start on healthy teeth.

4 cups	water or Vegetable Stock (see recipe, page 201) or Roasted Chicken Stock (see recipe, page 202)	1 L
1 cup	coarse cornmeal, preferably stone-ground (see Tips, left)	250 mL
½ cup	finely chopped broccoli florets	125 mL
½ cup	shredded extra-old Cheddar cheese	125 mL

1. In a saucepan, bring water to a boil over medium heat. Slowly pour cornmeal into the water while whisking constantly to avoid lumps. Cook, whisking, until cornmeal begins to "bloom" (see Tips, left) and the mixture starts to thicken, 3 to 4 minutes. Reduce heat to low and cook, whisking constantly, until mixture is thick, about 10 minutes.

2. Stir in broccoli and cheese. Cover saucepan, remove from heat and set aside until broccoli is fork tender and polenta is soft, about 30 minutes. Let cool until warm to the touch or refrigerate for up to 3 days.

Nutrients per serving (½ cup/125 mL)	
Calories 73	Dietary fiber . . . . . . 1.2 g
Protein . . . . 2.0 g	Sodium . . . . . . 260.2 mg
Total fat . . . . 1.0 g	Calcium . . . . 76.3 mg
Saturated fat. . . . . . 0.5 g	Iron . . . . 1.3 mg
Carbohydrates. . . . 14.7 g	Vitamin C. . . . . . . 5.0 mg

Not just for babies
A pinch of kosher salt and freshly ground pepper with about ¼ cup (50 mL) chopped green onions makes this dish a little more grown up.

Israeli Couscous with Grated Carrots and Chives

Chef Gianni Respinto first introduced Israeli couscous to me while I was training at Florida's East City Grill. This semolina flour pasta is much larger than regular couscous and is cooked like a risotto, although it has the texture of noodles. I know you and your baby will love it. It is usually found where rice is sold.

Makes about 2 cups (500 mL)

■ ■ ■

Chef Jordan's Tips

I prefer to use grated, not sliced, carrots in this recipe. Grating releases the water in carrots, which combines with the natural starch in the couscous to create a very creamy texture.

Nutrition Tip

Extra virgin olive oil is a richer source of polyphenols than regular olive oil or other refined oils. Polyphenols have both antioxidant and anti-inflammatory properties. Because it loses nutrients with exposure to heat and light, extra virgin olive oil should be in opaque or dark tinted glass in a dark, cool place away from heat (not above your stove).

1 tbsp	extra virgin olive oil	15 mL
1 cup	Israeli couscous	250 mL
2 cups	water or Vegetable Stock (see recipe, page 201)	500 mL
1/3 cup	grated peeled carrots	75 mL
1/4 cup	chopped chives	50 mL

1. In a saucepan, heat oil over medium heat. Add couscous and toast, stirring constantly, until golden brown, about 2 minutes. Add water and bring to a boil. Reduce heat to low and simmer until couscous is soft and water has evaporated, about 10 minutes. Stir in carrots and chives. Cool until warm to the touch or transfer to an airtight container and refrigerate for up to 3 days.

Nutrients per serving (1/2 cup/125 mL)	
Calories 80	Dietary fiber . . . . . . 0.9 g
Protein . . . . 1.7 g	Sodium . . . . 12.1 mg
Total fat . . . . 3.7 g	Calcium . . . . 12.3 mg
Saturated fat. . . . . . 0.5 g	Iron . . . . 0.2 mg
Carbohydrates. . . . 10.1 g	Vitamin C. . . . . . . 2.0 mg

Not just for babies
This recipe is certainly not just for babies. Bon appetit, Mom and Dad!

Jasmine Rice with Butternut Squash and Saffron

Jasmine rice is one of the most aromatic grains on the planet, and it's a breeze to cook, too! I've always found the texture of jasmine rice to be child friendly. It's soft and easy for kids to chew.

Makes about 2¼ cups (550 mL)

▪ ▪ ▪

Chef Jordan's Tips

This is a great method for achieving perfect rice every time. Just be sure not to lift the lid until the 20 minutes are up.

"Steep," in this case, refers to the infusion of the saffron cooking liquid into the rice. This combination is heavenly.

Nutrition Tip

Since ancient Egypt, saffron has been thought to have a calming effect on babies. It acts as an antispasmodic and cough suppressant, improves digestion and decreases gas. More recently, studies have demonstrated that this ancient spice may have anti-cancer and heart-protective properties.

1 tsp	unsalted butter	5mL
1 cup	finely diced peeled butternut squash	250 mL
1¼ cups	water or Vegetable Stock (see recipe, page 201)	300 mL
⅔ cup	jasmine rice, rinsed	150 mL
Pinch	saffron threads	Pinch

1. In a saucepan, melt butter over medium heat. Add squash and sauté until starting to soften, about 2 minutes. Stir in water, rice and saffron and bring to a boil. Cover, reduce heat to low and simmer for 5 minutes.

2. Remove from heat and let steep, covered, until liquid is absorbed and rice is tender, about 20 minutes. Let cool until warm to the touch or transfer to an airtight container and refrigerate for up to 2 days.

Nutrients per serving (½ cup/125 mL)	
Calories 78	Dietary fiber . . . . . . 1.3 g
Protein . . . . 1.4 g	Sodium . . . . 4.4 mg
Total fat . . . . 0.9 g	Calcium . . . . 29.3 mg
Saturated fat. . . . . . 0.6 g	Iron . . . . 0.5 mg
Carbohydrates. . . . 16.7 g	Vitamin C. . . . . . 11.8 mg

Not just for babies

This makes an excellent accompaniment to grilled skinless chicken breast. Bon appetit.

Whole-Grain Oat Crêpes with Warm Bananas

This delicious dish is a cross between crêpes and pancakes. Either way, these crêpes are amazing, and good for you, too!

Makes about 5 crêpes

∎ ∎ ∎

Chef Jordan's Tips

Breakfast casserole! Preheat the oven to 300°F (150°C). In a baking dish, layer the crêpes with fruit preserves. Once complete, pour 4 cups (1 L) whole milk whisked with 5 eggs over top to cover. Bake in preheated oven until firm, for 15 to 20 minutes. Garnish with freshly grated cinnamon.

1 cup	whole milk	250 mL
3	eggs	3
½ cup	old-fashioned rolled oats	125 mL
2 tsp	granulated sugar	10 mL
6 tbsp	whole wheat flour	90 mL
1 tsp	baking powder	5 mL
1 tbsp	unsalted butter, divided	15 mL
1	large banana, sliced	1

1. In a bowl, whisk together milk, eggs, oats and sugar. Whisk in flour and baking powder until moistened. Cover and refrigerate for at least 1 hour or overnight.

2. In a nonstick skillet, melt 1 tsp (5 mL) butter over medium heat. Ladle ½ cup (125 mL) of batter into the pan, swirling around to evenly coat the bottom of the pan. Cook until bottom is golden brown, 2 to 3 minutes. Flip and cook second side until light golden, about 1 minute. Transfer to a plate and repeat with remaining batter, adding more butter to the pan as necessary. Let cool until warm to the touch.

3. In the same skillet, cook sliced bananas over low heat until warm, about 2 minutes. Spoon over crêpes and let cool until warm to the touch.

Nutrients per serving			
Calories	209	Dietary fiber	3.5 g
Protein	9.1 g	Sodium	169.4 mg
Total fat	7.9 g	Calcium	102.7 mg
Saturated fat	3.4 g	Iron	1.7 mg
Carbohydrates	27.3 g	Vitamin C	2.4 mg

Not just for babies

Mom and Dad, how about serving these crêpes with a selection of fillings as a special dessert for your next dinner party? On a platter, layer the crêpes in the middle, surrounded by such toppings as vanilla-scented whipped cream, chocolate curls, ice cream, hazelnut spread — the options are endless. This dessert will knock their socks off, and I guarantee your guests will be talking about it for weeks to come!

Nutrition Tip

Whole grains are an important part of a healthy diet for you and your baby. Because they are minimally processed, they contain significant amounts of fiber, protein, essential oils, vitamins and minerals. Read your labels carefully to make sure you are actually getting whole grains. Canadians need to be particularly vigilant when purchasing whole wheat products, because the government has allowed flour that contains only 30 per cent of the germ to be labeled "whole wheat." Make sure the label says 100 per cent whole-grain whole wheat, to ensure you are getting the real thing.

French Toast with Fresh Peaches and Peachy Maple Syrup

When fresh peaches are in season, could there be a better way to start your family's day?

Makes about
6 servings

■ ■ ■

Chef Jordan's Tips

Be sure to use a brand of vanilla extract that doesn't contain alcohol.

If you don't have whole wheat bread, substitute challah or egg bread. The texture is a little softer and the finished product is more moist than whole wheat.

Use whatever is fresh and/or local in place of the peaches, such as apples, apricots or blueberries.

3	eggs	3
¼ cup	whole milk	50 mL
1 tsp	granulated sugar	5 mL
1 tsp	pure vanilla extract (see Tips, left)	5 mL
6	slices whole wheat bread	6
1 tbsp	unsalted butter, divided	15 mL
¼ cup	pure maple syrup	50 mL
1 cup	sliced pitted peaches	250 mL

1. In a bowl, whisk together eggs, milk, sugar and vanilla.

2. In a nonstick skillet, melt butter over medium heat. Working with 2 slices at a time, dip bread into egg mixture and place in the pan. Cook until bottom is golden brown, 2 to 3 minutes. Flip and cook until second side is golden brown, about 2 minutes. Transfer to a plate and repeat with remaining bread and egg mixture, adding more butter to the pan as necessary. Let cool until warm to the touch.

3. In the same skillet, over low heat, warm maple syrup, stirring constantly, for about 30 seconds. Spoon peach slices over French toast and drizzle with warm syrup. Extra French toast can be wrapped in plastic and refrigerated for up to 3 days.

Nutrients per serving	
Calories 168	Dietary fiber . . . . . . 2.4 g
Protein . . . . 6.3 g	Sodium . . . . . . 199.6 mg
Total fat . . . . 5.5 g	Calcium . . . . 31.3 mg
Saturated fat. . . . . . 2.1 g	Iron . . . . 1.3 mg
Carbohydrates. . . . 25.4 g	Vitamin C. . . . . . . 1.8 mg

Not just for babies

Another recipe the entire family can enjoy.

Nutrition Tip

Maple syrup contains several essential minerals, which makes it particularly appealing as a sweetener. It provides manganese, which helps your body produce energy, and zinc, which helps to keep the immune system strong. Although some believe darker syrups have a more intense concentration of vitamins and minerals, the grades have more to do with when the trees are tapped than with the nutrients they contain. The lightest syrups are from the earliest part of the season. The syrup darkens as the season progresses. Be careful of syrups labeled "maple-flavored" because they generally contain corn syrup or high-fructose corn syrup, which is very taxing on the liver and should be avoided completely.

Buy organic peaches

World's Best "Fish Sticks"

If turbot isn't available, Dover sole or halibut substitute very well.

Makes about 2 servings

■ ■ ■

Chef Jordan's Tips

Panko bread crumbs are coarser than regular bread crumbs and they tend to achieve a better crust. They are available in specialty food shops but if you can't find them, corn-flake crumbs make an excellent substitute.

Before serving any fish to a child, examine it closely for bones and remove any you find.

Nutrition Tip

Although your baby has not yet developed a taste for salt, if you do decide to use salt make sure you use it for taste and nutrition. We recommend using sea salt, which contains a smattering of many minerals, unlike refined table salt, which is virtually pure sodium chloride. Refined table salt also contains additives to prevent clumping.

1 cup	Panko bread crumbs (see Tips, left)	250 mL
1/3 cup	freshly grated Parmesan cheese	75 mL
1	egg white	1
1 tsp	water	5 mL
2 tbsp	extra virgin olive oil	25 mL
1	turbot fillet (about 8 oz/250 g)	1
1/2 cup	Caper and Lemon Remoulade (see recipe, page 207)	125 mL

1. In a bowl, combine bread crumbs and Parmesan cheese. Set aside. In another bowl whisk together egg white and water. Set aside.

2. Cut fillet into 10 "fingers" and toss into egg mixture to fully coat. One finger at a time, drain off most of the egg wash and toss into bread crumbs, pressing into crumbs. Repeat until all fingers are coated.

3. In a nonstick skillet, heat oil over medium heat. Add fish, in batches as necessary, and cook until golden brown on the bottom, about 2 minutes. Flip and cook until second side is golden brown and fish flakes easily with a fork, about 2 minutes. Let cool until warm to the touch. Serve with remoulade.

Nutrients per serving			
Calories	947	Dietary fiber	0.4 g
Protein	30.3 g	Sodium	1019.8 mg
Total fat	68.3 g	Calcium	174 mg
Saturated fat	9.3 g	Iron	3.1 mg
Carbohydrates	50.6 g	Vitamin C	4.5 mg

Not just for babies
The first time I tested this recipe for Jonah, I ate the whole thing myself.

Know Your Suppliers

In my world both Mom and Dad work full-time. With some planning, Tamar, Jonah and I manage to eat nutritious, delicious food Monday through Sunday. Sure, it's a little easier for me because of my background in the culinary world, but my wife has no training as a chef. However, she has become a wonderful cook in her own right, and one of the reasons is that she learned to let knowledgeable people guide the meals she cooks. She became acquainted with the staff at our local markets and questions them about what they are selling. They tell her what ingredients are the freshest and/or the best and she takes their advice when making decisions. If you get to know your local shop owners, they'll look out for you and make sure you are getting their very best products.

I think she learned this from me because I always try to develop relationships with my suppliers. Take my fishmonger, Gus. On the day I went looking for a flat fish to use in this recipe, Gus suggested turbot because it was the best fish he had. If turbot isn't available on the day you're trying this, ask your supplier the same question. You may end up with something else, but if he knows his stuff, with a little love, your dish will be great!

Alaskan Halibut en Papillote

The delicate flavor of the halibut shines through in this recipe and complements the fennel and sweet peppers. This recipe is super good.

Makes about 2 servings

■ ■ ■

Chef Jordan's Tips

Egg whites and yolks are typically combined with milk or water and brushed on pastries or breads to help create a golden brown color. In this instance, the egg whites combined with water act as the "glue" sealing the two edges of the parchment paper together.

For a unique serving idea, bring the package to the table, cut with scissors to open the paper and allow the kids to eat from the paper. It adds an element of fun to their dinner.

Remember, before serving any fish to a child, examine it closely for bones and remove any you find.

- Preheat oven to 300°F (150°C)
- 2 sheets parchment paper
- Baking sheet

½ cup	sliced fresh fennel	125 mL
⅓ cup	coarsely chopped asparagus	75 mL
⅓ cup	thin strips red bell pepper	75 mL
⅓ cup	thin strips yellow bell pepper	75 mL
1 tbsp	chopped chives	15 mL
1 tbsp	freshly squeezed lemon juice	15 mL
8 oz	Alaskan halibut fillet, cut into 2 pieces	250 g
1 tbsp	unsalted butter, divided	15 mL
1	egg white	1
1 tsp	water	5 mL

1. In a bowl, combine fennel, asparagus, red and yellow peppers, chives and lemon juice.

2. Fold 2 pieces of parchment paper, each approximately 12-by 8-inches (30 x 20 cm). Set one aside. Place half the vegetables on one side of one piece of parchment, place one piece of fish on top of the vegetables and top with half the butter. Fold the other side of the paper over to enclose the filling and twist the two ends, like a candy wrapper to create a seal. Repeat with remaining parchment, vegetables, fish and butter.

3. In a small bowl, whisk egg white with water. Brush the unsealed edges of the packages with the mixture, gluing them together (see Tips, left).

4. Place packages on a baking sheet and bake in preheated oven until paper turns golden brown, about 25 minutes. Let cool for 5 to 10 minutes before opening package. If necessary, let cool until warm to the touch before serving.

Nutrients per serving			
Calories	209	Dietary fiber	1.9 g
Protein	26.5 g	Sodium	131.4 mg
Total fat	9.3 g	Calcium	47.6 mg
Saturated fat	4.5 g	Iron	1.2 mg
Carbohydrates	6.2 g	Vitamin C	81.7 mg

Not just for babies

When I first attempted this recipe, I couldn't believe the depth of flavor the addition of fennel and lemon juice added to the halibut. This recipe would easily impress any adult, not just kids. To garnish the adult version, pick the fennel fronds from the stalk and sprinkle on top just before serving, adding a fresh dimension to the dish.

Nutrition Tip

Halibut is the highest animal source of magnesium, a mineral that supports every function in your baby's body. Magnesium partners with calcium to keep your baby's muscles and organs relaxed and healthy, helping to alleviate muscle cramps or sleeplessness. This mineral also helps relieve constipation.

Salmon, Potato and Cauliflower

Salmon and potato is a classic combination. The cauliflower adds textural contrast. It's a great way to introduce your toddler to this flavorful fish.

- Potato masher

3 cups	water	750 mL
1½ cups	coarsely chopped peeled russet potatoes	375 mL
1	piece (about 6 oz/175 g) skinless salmon fillet	1
⅔ cup	chopped cauliflower florets	150 mL

1. In a saucepan, combine water, potatoes, salmon and cauliflower. Bring to a boil over medium heat. Reduce heat to low and simmer until potatoes are fork tender, about 7 minutes.

2. In a colander set over a bowl, strain potato mixture, reserving cooking liquid. Transfer solids to a bowl. Add 2 cups (500 mL) of reserved cooking liquid. Using a potato masher, mash until smooth. Let cool until warm to the touch or transfer to an airtight container and refrigerate for up to 3 days or freeze for up to 1 month.

Nutrients per serving (½ cup/125 mL)	
Calories 138	Dietary fiber . . . . . . 2.3 g
Protein . . . . 10.7 g	Sodium . . . . 36.7 mg
Total fat . . . . 4.8 g	Calcium . . . . 33.3 mg
Saturated fat. . . . . . 0.8 g	Iron . . . . 1.0 mg
Carbohydrates. . . . 12.8 g	Vitamin C. . . . . . 35.5 mg

Not just for babies

Using the refrigerated mixture, form small patties. Bread in corn-flake or panko crumbs and in a nonstick skillet over medium heat, cook, turning once, until golden.

Pacific Salmon Cakes

I remember the salmon "patties" my mom used to make, which consisted of canned salmon with mayonnaise. Now I prefer to use Pacific wild salmon. Make extra when you're cooking salmon and save the leftovers to make this recipe.

Makes 6 cakes

■ ■ ■

Chef Jordan's Tips
Remember, before serving any fish to a child, examine it closely for bones and remove any you find.

Nutrition Tip
Salmon is one of the richest and best utilized sources of omega-3 fatty acids. These fats have many benefits, among which are their anti-inflammatory properties. Studies suggest that consuming good amounts of omega-3 fats throughout childhood and as an adult may decrease the risk of inflammatory and autoimmune diseases such as rheumatoid arthritis, Crohn's disease and multiple sclerosis.

Buy organic peppers

1 lb	cooked Pacific salmon fillet, skin removed and flaked	500 g
1/3 cup	diced red onion	75 mL
1/3 cup	fresh roasted corn kernels (see recipe, page 136)	75 mL
1/3 cup	diced red bell pepper	75 mL
1 tbsp	unsalted butter	15 mL

1. In a bowl, combine salmon, onion, corn and red pepper until well mixed. Form into six cakes, each about $1\frac{1}{2}$ inches (4 cm) thick. Place on a plate, cover and refrigerate until set, at least 1 hour or for up to 12 hours.

2. In a nonstick skillet, melt butter over medium-low heat. Add the cakes and cook until golden brown, about 5 minutes. Flip and cook until second side is golden brown, about 5 minutes. Transfer to a plate and let cool until warm to the touch or cover and refrigerate for up to 3 days.

Nutrients per serving (1 cake)	
Calories 182	Dietary fiber . . . . . . 0.5 g
Protein . . . . 17.0 g	Sodium . . . . 51.3 mg
Total fat . . . . 11.1 g	Calcium . . . . 13.4 mg
Saturated fat. . . . . . 3.0 g	Iron . . . . 0.4 mg
Carbohydrates. . . . . 2.9 g	Vitamin C. . . . . . 15.0 mg

Not just for babies
Serve these salmon cakes on a bed of Boston or "butter" lettuce with a simple dressing of fresh lemon juice, olive oil and minced garlic.

Classic Beef and Barley Stew

There's nothing better than the classics! These dishes become classics because they have universal appeal. Once your children taste this, I guarantee it will become a family favorite.

Makes about 5 cups (1.25 L)

◾ ◾ ◾

Chef Jordan's Tips

Browning or caramelizing meats is the essence of building flavors. After searing, fond develops on the bottom of the pan. Adding liquid and scraping the bits of fond into it, with a wooden or rubber utensil, develops the depth of flavor you want. For added flavor use vegetable stock instead of water.

• Potato masher, optional

2 tbsp	extra virgin olive oil	25 mL
1¼ cups	diced stewing beef	300 mL
¾ cup	barley	175 mL
¼ cup	diced sweet onion	50 mL
5 cups	water or Vegetable Stock (see recipe, page 201)	1.25 L
2	sprigs fresh thyme	2

1. In a saucepan, heat oil over medium heat. Add beef and sauté until golden brown, about 3 minutes. Add barley and onion and sauté until barley is golden brown, about 5 minutes.

2. Add water and thyme and bring to a boil. Reduce heat to low and simmer until beef and barley are tender and most of the water has evaporated, about 1½ hours. (If you're using whole barley, it should be tender at this point, but may need to be cooked longer.) Mash or cut to desired consistency. Let cool until warm to the touch or transfer to an airtight container and refrigerate for up to 3 days or freeze for up to 1 month.

Nutrients per serving (½ cup/125 mL)

Calories	67	Dietary fiber	0.5 g
Protein	2.7 g	Sodium	9.6 mg
Total fat	4.6 g	Calcium	7.2 mg
Saturated fat	1.1 g	Iron	0.5 mg
Carbohydrates	3.6 g	Vitamin C	0.5 mg

Not just for babies

A simple reduction of red wine will make an already fabulous dish even better. Before mashing, spoon off an appropriate quantity for your baby and add this reduction to the remainder. In a saucepan, over high heat, bring 1 cup (250 mL) of red wine to a boil and reduce by half.

Nutrition Tip

Red meat is one of the richest sources of vitamin B_{12}, which is found only in animal products and fermented foods. This vitamin affects the workings of your baby's nervous system and is essential for the production of red blood cells. If your baby is deficient in B_{12}, she may develop megaloblastic anemia, which can lead to neurological damage.

Fennel and Apple-Stuffed Pork Chops

This is a classic pairing of apples and pork — enjoy.

Makes about 2 servings

■ ■ ■

Chef Jordan's Tips

If you're serving this to children, refrigerate any leftovers for up to 3 days. To serve, dice finely, add a little water or chicken stock and reheat. Let cool until warm to the touch before serving.

- Preheat oven to 400°F (200°C)
- Ovenproof skillet

1 tsp	unsalted butter	5 mL
1 cup	finely diced cored apple	250 mL
¼ cup	finely diced fresh fennel	50 mL
2	bone-in pork chops (about 1 lb/500 g)	2
½ cup	fine cornmeal, preferably stone-ground	125 mL
1 tbsp	extra virgin olive oil	15 mL

1. In a skillet, melt butter over medium heat. Add apple and fennel and sauté until fennel is soft, about 5 minutes. Transfer to a bowl and let cool to room temperature, about 15 minutes.

2. On a cutting board, using a paring knife, make a small incision in the side of each pork chop opposite the bone, cutting toward the bone, right into the middle of the meat to create a pocket. Using your fingers, work the opening, making it as large as possible without tearing the meat (if you do it's not the end of the world).

3. Stuff pork chops with apple mixture and pinch the opening closed. On a plate, spread cornmeal evenly and thoroughly coat both sides of the pork chops. Discard any excess cornmeal.

4. In an ovenproof skillet, heat oil over medium heat. Add pork chops and sear until bottom is golden brown, about 5 minutes. Flip pork chops over and transfer the skillet to the preheated oven. Bake until just a hint of pink remains in pork, about 10 minutes. Cut a piece off and dice finely to serve to your baby, allowing to cool to room temperature before serving. Enjoy the remainder yourselves.

Nutrients per serving			
Calories	610	Dietary fiber	7.1 g
Protein	44.9 g	Sodium	847.3 mg
Total fat	31.9 g	Calcium	51.9 mg
Saturated fat	10.4 g	Iron	2.6 mg
Carbohydrates	35.5 g	Vitamin C	7.8 mg

Not just for babies

To put it into perspective, the first time I tested this recipe, Tamar and I cooked it for ourselves and shared it with Jonah. We enjoyed it as a family and I regretted not making more.

Nutrition Tip

Increasing levels of air pollution in North America are contributing to more children's respiratory issues. Fresh fennel (and even more so, fennel tea) will help relax bronchial passageways and is good for asthma, bronchitis and cough. A vegetable with many talents, fennel stimulates appetite — helpful if you are a parent of a finicky little eater.

Pork with Red Cabbage

This is a perfect flavor combination. I'm certain you and your baby will love it, too.

**Makes about
1¼ cups (300 mL)**

■ ■ ■

Chef Jordan's Tips

I have a real affinity for the combination of dried cherries with pork, but in the absence of dried cherries, most dried fruits would work well: currants, raisins, even apricots.

Nutrition Tip

Adequate amounts of vitamin A in your baby's body will ensure that her delicate skin has the greatest ability to rejuvenate and heal itself. Red cabbage is loaded with this vitamin and can help protect the skin from eczema and other rashes.

- Preheat oven to 350°F (180°C)
- Ovenproof skillet

1 tbsp	extra virgin olive oil	15 mL
8 oz	pork tenderloin	250 g
¾ cup	sliced red cabbage	175 mL
⅓ cup	dried cherries	75 mL
2	sprigs fresh thyme	2
¼ cup	water	50 mL

1. In ovenproof skillet, heat oil over medium-high heat. Add tenderloin and brown. Turn over pork. Add cabbage, cherries, thyme and water.

2. Roast in preheated oven until internal temperature of pork is 160°F (71°C), about 10 minutes. Mash or cut your baby's portion to desired consistency. Let cool until warm to the touch or transfer to an airtight container and refrigerate for up to 3 days.

Nutrients per serving (½ cup/125 mL)	
Calories 236	Dietary fiber . . . . . . 5.0 g
Protein . . . . 21.8 g	Sodium . . . . 57.8 mg
Total fat . . . . 9.1 g	Calcium . . . . 25.7 mg
Saturated fat. . . . . . 2.0 g	Iron . . . . 1.9 mg
Carbohydrates. . . . 15.3 g	Vitamin C. . . . . . 16.1 mg

Not just for babies

This is another one of those recipes that is absolutely perfect for the entire family as is, no additions necessary. Just mash a portion for Baby and serve the rest to Mom and Dad.

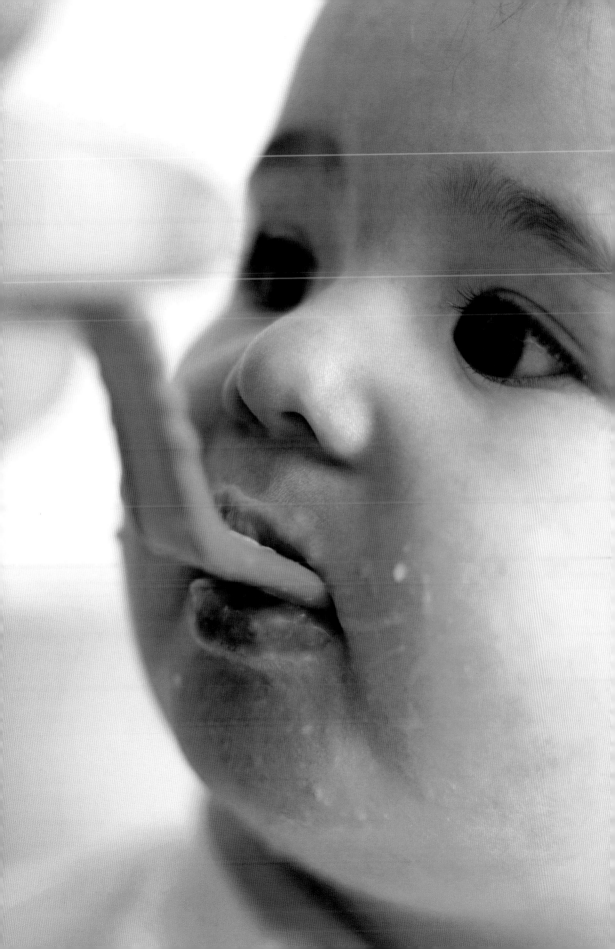

Roasted Summer Fruit (page 120) and Roasted Summer Fruit Smoothie (page 121)

French Toast with Fresh Peaches and
Peachy Maple Syrup (page 148)

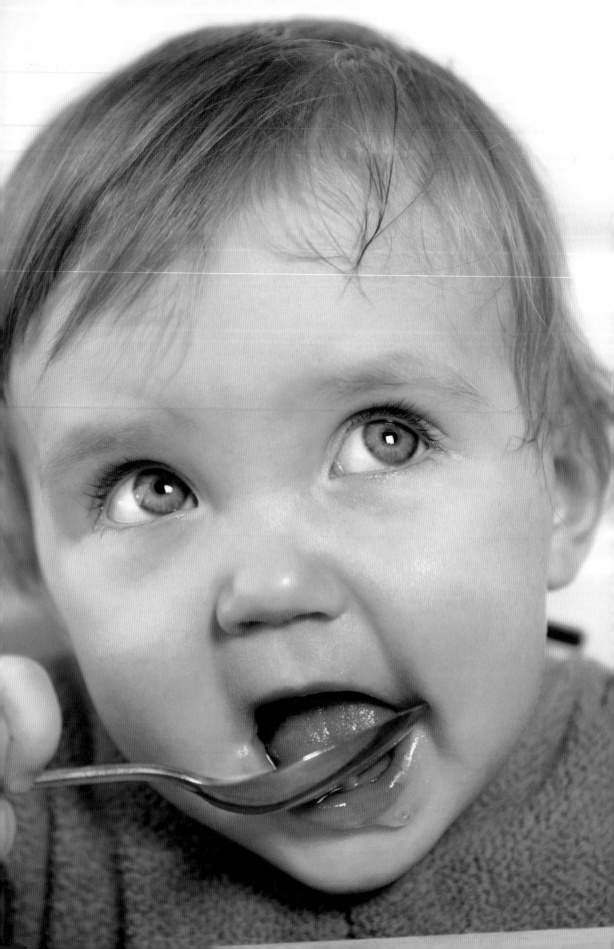

Fresh Herb-Crusted Veal Chops

This is a great meal for the children and you to enjoy together.

**Makes about
2 cups (500 mL)
diced or 2 adult
servings**

■ ■ ■

Chef Jordan's Tips

Although I always
recommend using fresh
herbs, this is one time
when I'll throw caution
to the wind and suggest
you use what you
and your family like,
whether fresh or dried.
Dried oregano, thyme
or parsley, or even a
combination of any or
all of these will result in
a very tasty veal chop.

Nutrition Tip

Veal is very low in
saturated fat and is
considered extra lean
when compared with
other meats such as
pork, chicken or beef.
Not only is it very rich
in protein to help keep
your baby's immune
system functioning
properly, but there are
also considerable
amounts of B_{12}, iron
and zinc, all of which
are important for
normal growth and
development.

- Preheat oven to 350°F (180°C)
- Ovenproof skillet

1 cup	bread crumbs, preferably panko	250 mL
1 tbsp	chopped fresh herbs (see Tips, left)	15 mL
1	egg	1
1 tbsp	whole milk	15 mL
1 tsp	unsalted butter	5 mL
2	veal chops (about 1 lb/500 g)	2

1. In a shallow bowl, combine bread crumbs and herbs. In another shallow bowl, whisk together egg and milk. Dip veal chops into egg mixture, then into bread crumbs, pressing to coat thoroughly. Place on a plate.

2. In an ovenproof skillet, melt butter over medium heat. Add veal chops and cook until golden brown on the bottom, 2 to 4 minutes. Flip veal chops over and transfer skillet to preheated oven. Bake until exterior is golden brown and meat is slightly pink inside, 10 to 12 minutes. Cut a piece off and dice finely to serve to your baby, allowing to cool to room temperature before serving.

Nutrients per adult serving	
Calories 516	Dietary fiber . . . . . . 2.0 g
Protein . . . . 54.4 g	Sodium . . . . . . 407.1 mg
Total fat . . . . 12.5 g	Calcium . . . . 67.9 mg
Saturated fat. . . . . . 4.4 g	Iron . . . . 3.0 mg
Carbohydrates. . . . 43.6 g	Vitamin C. . . . . . . 0.3 mg

Not just for babies
Mom and Dad, enjoy this meal, too!

Chicken with Caramelized Apples

Your children will absolutely adore the combination of chicken and butter with the sweetness of apples.

Makes about 1 cup (250 mL)

■ ■ ■

Chef Jordan's Tips

If ever you doubt your own instinct in determining whether a piece of chicken is cooked, remove the meat and cut in half to ensure that no hint of pink remains. When feeding babies and toddlers, it's best to take no chances, because any food-borne illness can have serious consequences.

Nutrition Tip

When selecting apples choose organic since the peel is so nutritionally vital. Do not wash apples before storing, but remove any soft or spoiled ones and keep the remainder loose and unbagged. Fruit gives off ethylene gas, which can take apples from crispy and fresh to soggy and old if they are stored in a bag.

Buy organic apples

1 tsp	unsalted butter	5 mL
2	diced boneless skinless chicken thighs, chopped (about 5 oz/150 g)	2
½ cup	chopped cored Gala or other sweet apple	125 mL
1⅓ cups	water	325 mL

1. In a saucepan, melt butter over medium heat. Add chicken and apple and sauté until apple is soft, about 5 minutes. Add water and bring to a boil. Reduce heat to low and simmer until juices run clear when chicken is pierced, 5 to 7 minutes (see Tips, left). Mash or cut to desired consistency.

2. Let cool until warm to the touch or transfer to an airtight container and refrigerate for up to 3 days or freeze for up to 1 month.

Nutrients per serving (½ cup/125 mL)	
Calories 139	Dietary fiber . . . . . . 1.5 g
Protein . . . . 14.9 g	Sodium . . . . 70.3 mg
Total fat . . . . 5.0 g	Calcium . . . . 16.7 mg
Saturated fat. . . . . . 2.0 g	Iron . . . . 0.9 mg
Carbohydrates. . . . . 8.6 g	Vitamin C. . . . . . . 2.9 mg

Not just for babies

Sorry, Mom and Dad. This recipe makes such a small quantity, it is just for babies.

Onion Soup with Cornish Hen

This twist on classic French onion soup is very simple and delicious.

Makes about 5 cups (1.25 L)

■ ■ ■

Chef Jordan's Tips

Cornish hen meat is similar to chicken in texture but not in flavor. I find these immature chickens have a more delicate and sweeter flavor than most free-range or more mature chickens. However, chicken is a little more readily available than Cornish hen and would certainly produce a wonderful soup for both you and your child.

Nutrition Tip

At about 12 months of age you will be starting to establish a food routine with your baby as you discover when he is the hungriest and when he needs to snack. It is normal to be concerned about how much your baby does or doesn't eat, but try to look at the bigger picture of his overall growth and weight rather than being overly concerned with the volume eaten in a particular day.

1 tbsp	unsalted butter	15 mL
3 cups	sliced white onions	750 mL
2	sprigs fresh thyme	2
2	cloves garlic, minced	2
4 cups	Roasted Chicken Stock (see recipe, page 202)	1 L
1 cup	shredded Cornish hen meat (see recipe, page 234)	250 mL

1. In a saucepan, melt butter over medium heat. Add onions, thyme and garlic and sauté until onions are soft, about 10 minutes.

2. Add chicken stock and Cornish hen and bring to a boil. Reduce heat to low and simmer until soup has reduced by one-quarter, about 10 minutes. Mash or cut your baby's portion to desired consistency. Let cool until warm to the touch or transfer to an airtight container and refrigerate for up to 3 days.

Nutrients per serving (½ cup/125 mL)	
Calories 148	Dietary fiber . . . . . . 1.7 g
Protein . . . . 10.4 g	Sodium . . . . 52.9 mg
Total fat . . . . 8.3 g	Calcium . . . . 33.9 mg
Saturated fat. . . . . . 2.7 g	Iron . . . . 0.8 mg
Carbohydrates. . . . . 7.9 g	Vitamin C. . . . . . . 7.9 mg

Not just for babies

This is another dish that Mom and Dad can enjoy right along with Baby.

Gramma Jean's Turkey Meatloaf

I lived with my Gramma Jean while attending culinary school in Ft. Lauderdale Fla. I owe this fan favorite to her (many of my customers throughout the years have raved about this recipe). I'm certain your baby will love it, too.

Makes about 8 servings

■ ■ ■

Chef Jordan's Tips

A few gentle taps of the loaf pan on your countertop will pack the meat tightly into the pan.

Brie cheese, a soft cow's milk cheese covered in a white rind, is one of my family's favorite cheeses. It makes a perfect addition to this meatloaf. As the cheese melts it seems to weave its way through the meat and is a wonderful flavor combination with the mushrooms and sweet peppers.

- Preheat oven to 300°F (150°C)
- 9-by 5-inch (2 L) loaf pan
- Instant-read thermometer

½ cup	diced whole wheat bread	50 mL
¼ cup	whole milk	50 mL
1 tsp	unsalted butter	5 mL
1½ cups	sliced mushrooms	375 mL
½ cup	finely diced red bell pepper	125 mL
1 lb	ground turkey	500 g
¼ cup	finely diced Brie cheese (rind on)	50 mL
1 tbsp	chopped basil leaves	15 mL

1. In a large bowl combine bread and milk; set aside until all the milk has soaked into the bread, 5 to 7 minutes.

2. In a skillet, melt butter over medium heat. Add mushrooms and sweet peppers and sauté until all liquid from mushrooms has evaporated, about 7 minutes. Transfer to the bowl with bread and let cool to room temperature.

3. Add turkey, Brie and basil to vegetable mixture and mix until combined. Pack into the loaf pan, ensuring there are no air pockets (see Tips, left).

4. Bake in preheated oven until thermometer inserted into center registers 165°F (75°C), about 45 minutes. Cut up to desired size. Let cool until warm to the touch, wrap in plastic wrap and refrigerate for up to 3 days.

Nutrients per serving			
Calories	132	Dietary fiber	0.9 g
Protein	13.1 g	Sodium	107.7 mg
Total fat	7.3 g	Calcium	44.2 mg
Saturated fat	2.6 g	Iron	1.0 mg
Carbohydrates	3.1 g	Vitamin C	12.9 mg

Not just for babies

Everyone in the family should enjoy this Wagman family classic together. Bon appetit.

Nutrition Tip

Why do we want to sleep after a turkey dinner? Turkey has high levels of tryptophan. This amino acid is the precursor to serotonin and melatonin, neurotransmitters that regulate vital functions of the central nervous system. Serotonin helps to keep you in a good mood, while melatonin calms the brain, settling your baby in to a peaceful night's sleep.

Oven-Roasted Duck Confit with Fresh Thyme

This recipe is so easy to make, yet it produces one of the most deliciously decadent dishes you'll ever eat.

Makes about 1 cup (250 mL)

■ ■ ■

Chef Jordan's Tips

Many gourmet food shops sell vacuum sealed, individually wrapped cooked duck legs. The work is already done for you, so there are no excuses.

Nutrition Tip

Many fresh herbs have long histories of medicinal use, and thyme is no exception. Thyme is a demulcent, which means it soothes irritated tissues, and an expectorant, which helps to clear phlegm and mucus from the air pathways. In fact, this herb is often used in cough mixtures. Thyme tea (1 tsp/5 mL dried thyme steeped for 10 minutes in 1 cup/ 250 mL boiling water) has traditionally been used to treat infected gums and sore throats.

- Preheat oven to 250°F (120°C)
- Ovenproof skillet

2	duck legs (about 1 lb/500 g)	2
2	sprigs fresh thyme	2

1. In ovenproof skillet over medium heat, sear duck legs, skin side down, until caramelized, about 10 minutes. Flip duck over and stir in thyme.

2. Bake in the preheated oven until meat is falling off the bone, about 2 hours. Let cool until warm to the touch. Pull meat off the bone, discarding skin and bones and shredding meat. Serve immediately, or transfer to an airtight container and refrigerate for up to 3 days.

Nutrients per serving (½ cup/125 mL)	
Calories 200	Dietary fiber . . . . . . 0.1 g
Protein . . . . 24.7 g	Sodium . . . . . . 101.3 mg
Total fat . . . . 10.5 g	Calcium . . . . 12.4 mg
Saturated fat. . . . . . 2.7 g	Iron . . . . 2.1 mg
Carbohydrates. . . . . 0.2 g	Vitamin C. . . . . . . 2.7 mg

Not just for babies

Mom and Dad will enjoy this recipe as is. Just add some vegetables of your choice.

Red Cabbage with Duck Confit

If you haven't tried duck confit, this French classic is easy to make and well worth the modest effort.

Makes about 1¼ cups (300 mL)

■ ■ ■

Chef Jordan's Tips

My favorite duck for making duck confit is Moulard duck, a cross between Peking and muscovy ducks. I often see frozen ducks in grocery stores. If thawed correctly, on a plate on the bottom shelf of the refrigerator over the course of a day or two, these are very good alternatives.

Nutrition Tip

This recipe makes a great dinner for both you and your child. The duck provides a rich protein source and the cabbage adds vitamins and minerals. To complete the picture, round it off with a nice single or mixed fruit purée. If you make enough, this would be a good leftover for your baby for lunch tomorrow paired with some soft cooked and chopped green beans or cauliflower florets.

- Potato masher, optional

1 tsp	unsalted butter	5 mL
2½ cups	sliced red cabbage	625 mL
1 cup	water	250 mL
½ cup	shredded cooked duck confit (see recipe, page 166)	125 mL
1 tsp	red wine vinegar	5 mL

1. In a saucepan, melt butter over medium heat. Add cabbage and sauté until wilted, about 2 minutes. Add water, duck and vinegar and bring to a boil. Reduce heat to low and simmer until cooking liquid has reduced by about three-quarters, about 6 minutes. Mash or cut to desired consistency. Let cool until warm to the touch or transfer to an airtight container and refrigerate for up to 3 days.

Nutrients per serving (½ cup/125 mL)	
Calories 92	Dietary fiber . . . . . . 1.5 g
Protein . . . . 7.6 g	Sodium . . . . 40.3 mg
Total fat . . . . 4.8 g	Calcium . . . . 38.3 mg
Saturated fat. . . . . . 2.2 g	Iron . . . . 1.3 mg
Carbohydrates. . . . . 5.2 g	Vitamin C . . . . 40 mg

Not just for babies

I could write this exact recipe for any cookbook and, with the exception of the mashing, virtually nothing would change. Everything about the dish is appropriate for Mom and Dad, so enjoy.

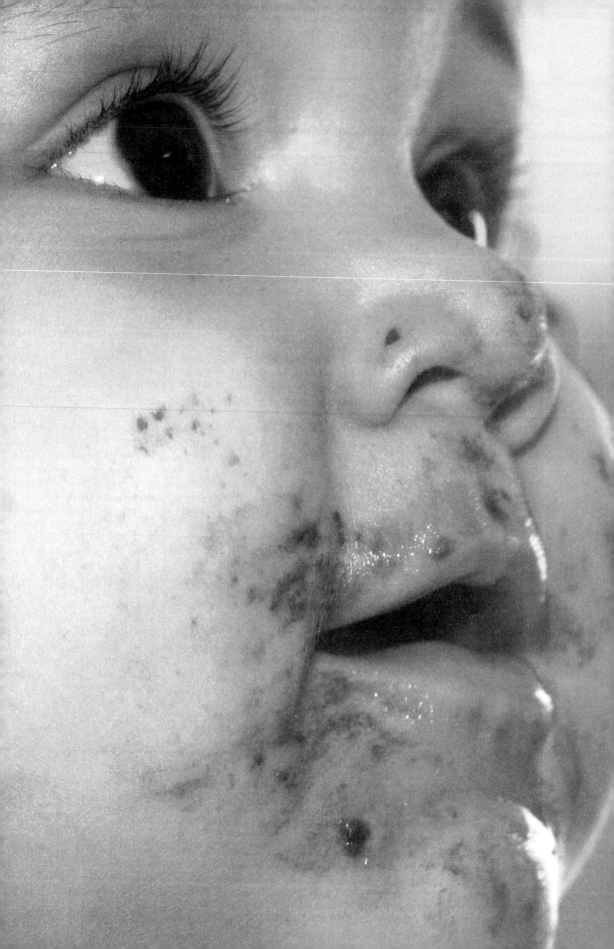

Snacks and Desserts

Introduction 170

Snacks

Sour Cream "Latkes" 172

Frozen Fruit Snacks. 173

"Chips and Salsa" — Parmesan
   Cheese Crisps with Plum Salsa . . 174

Chunky Pineapple Ice Pops 175

Mini Sweet Potato Muffins
   with Maple Syrup Glaze 176

Cheddar Cheese Dip. 178

Mini Chocolate Chunk Banana
   Sandwiches. 180

Guacamole. 182

Desserts

Frozen Blueberry Sorbet 183

Strawberries and Coconut Cream . . 184

My Mom's Applesauce 186

Frozen Mango Mousse 187

Chocolate Macaroons. 188

Pomegranate and Kiwi Purée
   with Crème Fraîche 189

Cheesecake Soufflé. 190

Maple Syrup-Glazed Pineapple 192

Short-Grain Brown Rice Pudding
   with Chocolate Wafers 193

Berry-Glazed Fig Tart 194

Cranberry Phyllo "Pinwheels" 195

Introduction

As we mentioned in Chapter 3, snacks are important for your toddler. They provide the added energy these busy little people need as they grow and develop. Snacking can expand the types of foods your child eats and can provide a way to ensure he gets the nutrients he needs if he hasn't eaten particularly well at mealtime. In fact, snacking, or "grazing," as some like to call it, is really the natural rhythm for toddlers.

The problem is, because it's convenient we often reach for snack foods that are heavy on sugar or full of processed grains, which don't have much to offer from a nutritional perspective. Worse still, there is reason to believe these foods may even contribute to childhood obesity. To keep your child on track, the trick is to offer snacks that are nutrient-dense. For instance, using the recipes from other sections of this book, consider offering your toddler pieces of soft sliced fruit to dip in Vanilla Bean Yogurt (see recipe, page 82), cooked vegetables or small pieces of whole wheat pita served with Fresh Soy Bean Hummus (see recipe, page 103) or even cold slices of Crispy Potato Galette (see recipe, page 132). In this chapter, we've provided recipes for snacks you can prepare for your child, but there are lots of other options you are likely to have on hand. Choose cooked whole grains, small pieces of cooked vegetables, soft fruits or protein, such as cubes of cheese or thin slices of chicken. These will help you provide your toddler with the nutrients he needs to make it from meal to meal.

Throughout this book we have provided you with recipes made from fresh whole foods, generally without sugar. But there is a time for everything. Our philosophy is that by making your own baby food you can control the ingredients you feed your child. Making dessert is no different. You can choose the juiciest most perfectly ripened fruit and you can determine how sweet you want the result to be.

We have used a variety of different types of sweeteners, from maple syrup to agave nectar, and have limited the use of granulated sugar. Sweet treats may be a bit of an indulgence, but they have a place in a well-balanced diet, just so long as they don't crowd out more healthful offerings, such as fresh fruits, vegetables and whole grains.

Sour Cream "Latkes"

This recipe evolved from my Gramma's loaded-with-sugar cheese latkes.

Makes about 25 cakes

■ ■ ■

Chef Jordan's Tips

This recipe demonstrates how, with a little thought and preparation, keeping your family on track for healthy eating is not all that difficult. These latkes freeze well and are simple to reheat. In a nonstick skillet, melt a little butter and sear the frozen cakes until warm, about 2 minutes.

Nutrition Tip

Using whole grains and their flours in your cooking dramatically increases the nutritional value of the finished dish. Refined grains can be stripped of as much as 90 per cent of their B vitamins, 70 per cent of their fiber, 70 per cent of their essential fatty acids and 60 per cent of their calcium. Refining does provide extra shelf life but at the sacrifice of a great deal of nutrition.

¾ cup	full-fat sour cream	175 mL
¼ cup	raw cane or granulated sugar	50 mL
2	eggs, beaten	2
1 tsp	pure vanilla extract	5 mL
⅓ cup	whole wheat, barley or buckwheat flour, sifted	75
1 tbsp	unsalted butter, divided	5 mL

1. In a bowl, whisk sour cream, sugar, eggs and vanilla. Gradually add flour, whisking until smooth.

2. In a nonstick skillet, melt ½ tsp (2 mL) of the butter over medium heat. Using 1 tbsp (15 mL) for each cake, spoon in batter in batches, keeping cakes separate. Cook until edges crisp, 2 to 3 minutes. Flip and cook until edges start to curl up toward the sky, about 1 minute. Repeat with remaining batter, adding more butter as necessary. Let cool to room temperature. Transfer to an airtight container and freeze for up to 6 months.

Nutrients per latke	
Calories 34	Dietary fiber . . . . . . 0.2 g
Protein . . . . 0.9 g	Sodium . . . . 13.3 mg
Total fat . . . . 2.0 g	Calcium . . . . 7.3 mg
Saturated fat. . . . . . 1.1 g	Iron . . . . 0.3 mg
Carbohydrates. . . . . 3.2 g	Vitamin C. . . . . . . 0.0 mg

Not just for babies

Frozen latkes are always great to have on hand. For brunch offer an assortment of preserves, peanut butter and maple syrup. In the evening provide smoked salmon, caramelized onions and an assortment of cheeses.

Frozen Fruit Snacks

Although it is extremely simple, small bits of frozen fruit make a great snack for kids and adults alike. Here we've provided the basic instructions for freezing grapes, but you can use them to make frozen berries, peaches, bananas, pineapple, kiwi or mango. Choose your family's favorite fruits — if they like to eat them fresh, just wait until they try them frozen.

**Makes about
1 lb (500 g)**

■ ■ ■

Nutrition Tip

One of the most healthful components of red grapes is the flavonoid resveratrol, which is found in their skins. Scientists are actively engaged in studying this compound, which may have a wide range of health benefits, from helping your body to fight viruses to increasing stamina. Red wine is another good source of resveratrol, so enjoy a glass while treating your children to their own source with frozen grape snacks.

Buy organic grapes

• Rimmed baking sheet lined with parchment paper

1 lb	seedless grapes	500 g

1. In a colander, under cold water, gently rinse the grapes and transfer to a paper towel to dry. Cut into halves or quarters, depending upon the age of your child. Place on the lined baking sheet and transfer to the freezer. Freeze until grapes are completely frozen, about 5 hours. Transfer to an airtight container and store frozen. Enjoy immediately or keep frozen for up to 6 months.

Nutrients per serving (¼ cup/50 mL)	
Calories 15	Dietary fiber . . . . . . 0.2 g
Protein . . . . 0.2 g	Sodium . . . . 0.0 mg
Total fat . . . . 0.2 g	Calcium . . . . 3.3 mg
Saturated fat. . . . . . 0.0 g	Iron . . . . 0.6 mg
Carbohydrates. . . . . 4.0 g	Vitamin C. . . . . . . 2.5 mg

Not just for babies

Frozen fruit is something adults can enjoy as a snack just as much as kids. Leave the fruit whole or cut it into larger pieces for the bigger folk. It also makes a great addition to salads or a pretty garnish for dessert. Often I serve frozen grapes as a dessert, along with a bowl of warm chocolate sauce for dipping.

"Chips and Salsa" — Parmesan Cheese Crisps with Plum Salsa

This is a scrumptious, healthy spin-off of my favorite snack, tortilla chips and tomato salsa. It's also a great way to get your kids to eat fruit.

Makes about 5 servings

■ ■ ■

Chef Jordan's Tips

This is the method restaurants use to create edible vessels like Parmesan "cannoli" or cups. The crisps remain pliable for a few moments after being removed from the heat, which provides time to mold them around a tube creating a cannoli shape, or over the outside of a ramekin to create a cup. Either way, it's an impressive way to serve appetizers.

Nutrition Tip

Plums and their dried version, prunes, have been studied for their unique phytochemicals, specifically neochlorogenic and chlorogenic acids. These nutrients help prevent damage to the important fats in our brain cells and cell membranes. On a more practical level, these fruits relieve constipation.

1½ cups	finely diced pitted plums	375 mL
1 tbsp	balsamic vinegar	15 mL
1 tbsp	liquid honey	15 mL
1 tsp	grated lemon zest	5 mL
1 cup	freshly grated Parmesan cheese	250 mL

1. In a bowl, combine plums, vinegar, honey and lemon zest. Set aside.

2. In a nonstick skillet over medium heat, spoon 1 tsp (5 mL) Parmesan cheese into the pan (per crisp) and cook until golden brown, about 3 minutes (be sure not to overload the pan as the cheese will melt and run together). Using a spatula, carefully transfer to a plate to cool. Repeat until all crisps are cooked. Once crisps are cooled, serve on a platter with a bowl of plum salsa.

Nutrients per serving	
Calories 115	Dietary fiber . . . . . . 0.0 g
Protein . . . . 6.8 g	Sodium . . . . . . 265.5 mg
Total fat . . . . 4.9 g	Calcium . . . . . . 196.2 mg
Saturated fat. . . . . . 2.9 g	Iron . . . . 0.2 mg
Carbohydrates. . . . 11.3 g	Vitamin C. . . . . . . 6.6 mg

Not just for babies

I've often served this exact hors d'oeuvre to guests. The saltiness of the cheese crisps combines with the sweetness of the fruit to create a delicious flavor contrast.

Chunky Pineapple Ice Pops

This is a very refreshing way to satisfy your child's cravings for sweets. And don't forget to have one yourself.

Makes about 14 ice pops

■ ■ ■

Chef Jordan's Tips

To make chunky pineapple purée, peel and core one medium pineapple. In a food processor or using an immersion blender, pulse until chunky. Retaining some texture creates an excellent contrast between the smooth ice and the chunky pineapple bits.

This recipe and can be used to make ice pops with most fruits, although some may require a little more sugar. Trust your palate.

Nutrition Tip

Making puréed fruits into ice pops is a creative way to increase the fruit in your child's diet. All fruits contain healthful vitamins and phytonutrients, such as flavonoids, that provide antioxidant protection to every cell in your baby's body.

- Popsicle sticks

1¼ cups	fresh chunky pineapple purée (about 1 medium pineapple) (see Tips, left)	300 mL
½ cup	water	125 mL
1 tbsp	agave nectar	15 mL

1. In a mixing bowl, combine pineapple, water and agave nectar. Mix thoroughly. Transfer to an ice cube tray and freeze just until surface has frozen, about 1 hour. Remove tray and cover tightly with plastic wrap. Using the tip of a sharp knife, pierce a small slit in the plastic directly over the middle of each cube. Insert the Popsicle sticks until they are submerged in the purée. Freeze until completely solid, about 2 hours. Although these will keep frozen for up to 1 month, I doubt they'll last that long.

Nutrients per ice pop	
Calories 15	Dietary fiber . . . . . . 0.9 g
Protein . . . . 0.3 g	Sodium . . . . 0.9 mg
Total fat . . . . 0.2 g	Calcium . . . . 3.9 mg
Saturated fat. . . . . 0.1 g	Iron . . . . 0.0 mg
Carbohydrates. . . . 3.5 g	Vitamin C. . . . . . . 4.4 mg

Not just for babies

Not just for babies, toddlers, teenagers or adults...this recipe is for the entire family to enjoy.

Mini Sweet Potato Muffins with Maple Syrup Glaze

Even though there is a minimal amount of sugar in these muffins (if you include the glaze; none if you omit it) they will delight your children. They will be begging you to make them, over and over again.

Makes about 36 muffins

■ ■ ■

Chef Jordan's Tips

What an excellent way to incorporate more vegetables into your children's diet. The muffins are completely sugar-free, so feel free to omit the glaze.

Be sure to use pure vanilla extract and make sure it's alcohol-free.

- Preheat oven to 300°F (150°C)
- 36-cup mini muffin tins, greased

Muffins

1 cup	unbleached all-purpose flour	250 mL
1 tsp	baking powder	5 mL
Pinch	kosher salt	Pinch
³⁄₄ cup	Roasted Sweet Potato Purée (see recipe, page 42)	175 mL
¹⁄₂ cup	agave nectar	125 mL
¹⁄₂ cup	whole milk	125 mL
1 tsp	melted unsalted butter	5 mL
1	whole egg	1
1 tsp	vanilla seeds (about 1 vanilla pod) or 1 tsp (5 mL) vanilla extract	5 mL

Glaze (optional)

¹⁄₂ cup	confectioner's (icing) sugar	125 mL
¹⁄₄ cup	Roasted Sweet Potato Purée (see recipe, page 42)	50 mL
1 tbsp	maple syrup	15 mL
1 tsp	milk	5 mL

1. In a bowl, whisk flour, baking powder and salt. Set aside.

2. In a separate bowl, whisk sweet potato, agave nectar, milk and melted butter until combined. Add egg and vanilla and whisk until integrated Fold dry ingredients into the wet, mixing just until incorporated. Do not overmix.

3. Spoon batter into prepared muffin tins until they are about two-thirds full. Bake in preheated oven until muffins have risen and a toothpick comes out clean when inserted into the center, about 10 minutes. Allow to cool until warm to the touch.

4. *Glaze, optional:* In a bowl, whisk together confectioner's sugar, purée, maple syrup and milk until glossy and thick. Cover and refrigerate until ready to use. When ready to serve, dip tops of the muffins into the glaze.

Nutrients per muffin			
Calories	28	Dietary fiber	0.2 g
Protein	0.7 g	Sodium	27.8 mg
Total fat	0.4 g	Calcium	9.3 mg
Saturated fat	0.2 g	Iron	0.2 mg
Carbohydrates	5.6 g	Vitamin C	0.1 mg

Not just for babies

Divide the batter into portions and use some to make larger "Mom and Dad-" size muffins. Just follow the recipe but use a 6- or 12-cup muffin tin and cook for about 20 minutes.

Nutrition Tip

These mini muffins are a healthy snack for your baby once he is old enough to enjoy small finger foods. Even though they are sweet, the ingredients can help keep blood sugar levels stable. The agave nectar contains fructose, which takes longer to break down into glucose (blood sugar) in the body than granulated sugar (sucrose). This means the blood sugar rises more slowly, putting less stress on the pancreas to release insulin. In addition, the roasted sweet potato purée provides soluble fiber, which also helps to keep blood sugar under control. For an extra dose of fiber, substitute an equal quantity of whole wheat flour for the all-purpose called for in this recipe.

Cheddar Cheese Dip

This is the greatest all-purpose cheese dip you and your children have ever tasted. At the Wagman household, we use this dip with just about everything, from vegetables and bread to sandwich meat and pizza.

Makes about 1 cup (250 mL)

∎ ∎ ∎

Chef Jordan's Tips

Vary this recipe to suit ingredients you have on hand. Make a simple "ratatouille" dip by adding 1 tbsp (15 mL) each of finely diced red bell pepper, yellow bell pepper, tomato and zucchini, immediately after you whisk the milk and flour together. Bring the vegetables to a simmer with the mixture and cook until it thickens.

Nutrition Tip

This is a great way to help ensure your child gets enough calcium. Not only is there ample calcium in the milk, cheese and yogurt, but the yogurt also contains intestine-friendly lactobacteria that help her body digest the calcium it contains, making it easier to absorb. This means even more calcium to build strong teeth and bones.

½ cup	milk	125 mL
1 tsp	unbleached all-purpose flour	5 mL
1 cup	grated Cheddar cheese	250 mL
½ cup	full-fat plain yogurt or sour cream	125 mL

1. In a saucepan over medium-low heat, bring milk and flour to a simmer, whisking constantly to prevent lumps. Continue whisking until mixture thickens, about 5 minutes. Remove from heat. Add cheese in small handfuls, whisking until fully melted and incorporated. Add yogurt and whisk to combine. Serve immediately or refrigerate for up to 3 days and serve chilled.

Nutrients per serving (¼ cup/50 mL)	
Calories 152	Dietary fiber . . . . . . 0.0 g
Protein . . . . 10.1 g	Sodium . . . . . . 218.1 mg
Total fat . . . . 10.4 g	Calcium . . . . . . 292.0 mg
Saturated fat . . . . . . 6.5 g	Iron . . . . 0.2 mg
Carbohydrates . . . . . 4.7 g	Vitamin C . . . . 0.0 mg

Not just for babies
Everyone in the family can enjoy this recipe as is.

All Fat Isn't Bad

Fat has gotten a bad rap in the past, but more and more research is showing us the benefits of different types of fat and how, despite the fact that it is high in calories, fat is an important component of a healthy diet. Without fat, for instance, your body would not be able to absorb the fat-soluble vitamins A, D, E and K.

Fat is made of building blocks called fatty acids, some of which are essential. For instance, your body needs omega-3 fats, found in fish such as salmon, cod, mackerel and herring, as well as some nuts and seeds. These fats have many benefits, such as reducing the risk of heart disease, contributing to good brain function and decreasing inflammation associated with degenerative diseases such as type-2 diabetes, and are in short supply in the typical North American diet. Omega-6 fats found in vegetable oils such as sunflower and safflower oils are also essential, but evidence is mounting that people who live in North America consume an excessive amount of these fats. Then there is saturated fat. Although much vilified, saturated fats are part of the building blocks for cell membranes and a variety of hormones and should be consumed in moderation. Trans fats that result from the process of partial hydrogenation are the exception. Many researchers believe there are no safe levels of consumption for these fats.

Just remember, though, that babies need proportionately more fat in their diet than adults. Avoid reduced-fat products when feeding your baby and ensure that there are good quantities of health promoting omega-3 fats in her diet.

Mini Chocolate Chunk Banana Sandwiches

This cake-like cookie tastes great by itself and works beautifully to create awesome snack sandwiches.

Makes about 18 cookies

■ ■ ■

Chef Jordan's Tips

Chocolate chips are a fine substitute for chunks but I love the inconsistency of the chunks — one bite is full of chocolate and the next bite, nothing. It keeps you coming back for more. To create chunks, buy baking chocolate that comes in small "bricks" at the grocery store and cut with a knife on a cutting board to achieve the desired consistency.

Be sure to use pure vanilla extract and make sure it is alcohol-free.

- Preheat oven to 350°F (180°C)
- Cookie sheet, lightly greased

2 cups	pastry flour	500 mL
½ tsp	baking powder	2 mL
Pinch	kosher salt	Pinch
1 cup	packed brown sugar	250 mL
¼ cup	unsalted butter, softened	50 mL
2	eggs	2
1 tsp	vanilla extract (or fresh vanilla beans from 1 pod)	5 mL
¼ cup	bittersweet chocolate chunks (see Tips, left)	50 mL
2	ripe bananas, peeled and thinly sliced	2

1. In a bowl, combine flour, baking powder and salt.

2. In a separate bowl, using an electric mixer on medium speed, beat brown sugar and butter until light and fluffy, about 3 minutes. Add eggs and vanilla, mixing until fully incorporated. On low speed, add dry ingredients, mixing just until combined. Stir in chocolate chunks.

3. Using two spoons to create a football shape, drop dough by heaping tablespoonfuls (15 mL) about 2 inches (5 cm) apart onto prepared cookie sheet. Bake in preheated oven until golden brown, about 15 minutes. Cool for 5 minutes on baking sheet then transfer to a rack and cool completely.

4. To make sandwiches, slice cookies in half across the "equator." Place a few slices of banana on one side and place the other half on top, enclosing the bananas. Serve immediately or freeze for up to 1 month.

Nutrients per cookie			
Calories	116	Dietary fiber	1.1 g
Protein	1.7 g	Sodium	34.3 mg
Total fat	3.9 g	Calcium	9.0 mg
Saturated fat	2.2 g	Iron	0.3 mg
Carbohydrates	20.0 g	Vitamin C	1.1 mg

Not just for babies

Well, folks, I guarantee you'll never have to purchase store-bought ice cream sandwiches again. Just follow the recipe but before closing the sandwich, scoop 1 tbsp (15 mL) vanilla ice cream onto the bananas. Enjoy one of the simplest pleasures around.

Nutrition Tip

One of the biggest benefits of making your own desserts and snacks is that you control the ingredients and know exactly what they contain. Many commercially prepared baked goods contain nutritionally inferior ingredients such as artificial flavors and colors, as well as preservatives designed to increase shelf life. With home baking you can avoid trans fats, which are found in most vegetable shortenings, as well as high-fructose corn syrup, which is increasingly linked with type-2 diabetes.

Guacamole

This is a staple in our home, whether served at snacktime with tortilla chips or with vegetables as a pre-dinner dip.

Makes about 2 cups (500 mL)

■ ■ ■

Chef Jordan's Tips

When storing guacamole in the refrigerator be sure to place a layer of plastic wrap directly on top of the mixture to prevent air from getting in, which will turn your avocado brown.

Nutrition Tip

Avocados contain the carotenoids lutein and zeaxanthin, both of which may help keep your baby's eyes healthy. Avocados also contain a significant amount of healthy monounsaturated fat. Carotenoids are fat-soluble, meaning that fat must be present for them to be absorbed. A recent study in the *Journal of Nutrition* demonstrated a significant improvement in the body's ability to absorb carotenoids from other vegetables when avocados were eaten at the same time.

¼ cup	chopped tomatoes	50 mL
1	minced green onion	1
1 tsp	fresh lemon juice	5 mL
2	avocados, peeled and pitted	2

1. In a mixing bowl combine tomatoes, green onion and lemon juice and mix well to combine. Add avocado and, using a fork, begin to break it up. Continue to mix until the desired consistency is achieved. Serve immediately or refrigerate for up to 3 days.

Nutrients per serving (¼ cup/50 mL)

Calories 82	Dietary fiber . . . . . . 3.5 g
Protein . . . . 1.1 g	Sodium . . . . 3.9 mg
Total fat . . . . 7.4 g	Calcium . . . . 7.6 mg
Saturated fat. . . . . . 1.1 g	Iron . . . . 0.3 mg
Carbohydrates. . . . . 4.7 g	Vitamin C. . . . . . . 6.7 mg

Not just for babies

Everyone loves guacamole. Enjoy!

Frozen Blueberry Sorbet

Puréed frozen blueberries, with the addition of agave nectar, taste like sorbet. You can serve this to your children instead of ice cream...you'll actually get away with it!

Makes about 1 lb (500 g)

◾ ◾ ◾

Chef Jordan's Tips

Make a double portion of the frozen berries and keep half on hand for snacks or as a garnish for watermelon soup, (see Not just for babies, below). Our family loves to eat frozen blueberries alone or added to our morning cereal.

Nutrition Tip

Blueberries are called a "super food" because they contain more antioxidants than virtually any other fruit or vegetable. If possible, feed them to your baby every day. Their high antioxidant level helps support your baby's immune system and, over time, reduces the risk of cancer and degenerative disease. Recent animal studies suggest blueberries might help brain cells communicate better and may actually encourage the brain to grow new cells. Brain food never tasted so good.

● Baking sheet, lined with parchment paper

| 2 cups | whole fresh blueberries | 500 mL |
| 1/4 cup | agave nectar | 50 mL |

1. In a colander, under cold water, gently rinse berries and transfer to a paper towel to thoroughly dry. Place on prepared baking sheet and transfer to the freezer, freezing until berries are completely frozen, about 5 hours.

2. Place frozen berries in a blender, in batches. Add agave nectar in batches and purée. Transfer to an airtight container and freeze. Before serving, remove the sorbet from the freezer to temper. Scrape with the tines of a fork to loosen the mixture or simply transfer to a blender for a quick purée. Enjoy immediately or freeze for up to 6 months.

Nutrients per serving (1/4 cup/50 mL)	
Calories 51	Dietary fiber . . . . . . 0.9 g
Protein . . . . 0.3 g	Sodium . . . . 0.4 mg
Total fat . . . . 0.1 g	Calcium . . . . 2.2 mg
Saturated fat. . . . . . 0.0 g	Iron . . . . 0.1 mg
Carbohydrates. . . . 13.4 g	Vitamin C. . . . . . . 3.4 mg

Not just for babies

A wonderful summer dessert is watermelon soup garnished with frozen blueberries and/or a dollop of blueberry sorbet. Just purée 2 cups (500 mL) seedless watermelon in a food processor with 1/4 cup (50 mL) agave syrup. Strain through a fine mesh strainer and garnish to your liking.

Strawberries and Coconut Cream

The contrast of textures — cold, hard strawberries and "pillow-like" whipping cream — make this a favorite anytime, but particularly on a warm summer day.

Makes 4 to
6 servings

■ ■ ■

Chef Jordan's Tips
When freezing fruit it's important not to stack the fruit because you're looking for individually frozen pieces. To prevent the individual pieces from sticking together or to the parchment paper, shake the baking sheet often while the berries are freezing.

Nutrition Tip
Strawberries are one of the foods most commonly associated with allergies, so we recommend you include strawberries in your baby's diet only after the first year, and then do so with caution. Introduce strawberries at a meal when you are not introducing any other new foods. This way you will be able to tell if there is an adverse reaction to the strawberries as opposed to any other new food.

- Baking sheet, lined with parchment paper

3 cups	hulled fresh strawberries	750 mL
1 cup	whipping (35%) cream	250 mL
1 tbsp	unsweetened shredded coconut, toasted	15 mL

1. In a colander, under cold water, gently rinse berries. Drain well and transfer to paper towel to dry. Cut strawberries into quarters and place on prepared baking sheet. Freeze until berries are completely frozen, about 5 hours. Transfer to an airtight container and freeze for up to 6 months.

2. In a mixing bowl, whisk (you can also do this using an electric mixer) cream until stiff peaks form. Add coconut and continue to whisk until fully combined. The cream can be refrigerated for up to 24 hours. Serve the strawberries and cream separately, using the cream as a dip.

Nutrients per serving	
Calories 248	Dietary fiber . . . . . . 2.4 g
Protein . . . . 2.0 g	Sodium . . . . 24.1 mg
Total fat . . . . 23.1 g	Calcium . . . . 56.2 mg
Saturated fat. . . . . 14.4 g	Iron . . . . 0.5 mg
Carbohydrates. . . . 10.2 g	Vitamin C. . . . . . 63.9 mg

Not just for babies
On a hot summer day, mix these berries and the coconut whipped cream with strands of mint and a dash of orange liqueur for a cool summer snack.

The Nose Knows

Raw Cane Sugar

When making desserts, we often like to use raw cane sugar, which is not as processed as granulated white sugar and retains some of the nutrients found in sugar cane. It is available in a number of forms such as Demerara, turbinado and muscovado, which vary in texture and flavor depending upon the molasses content.

I'm a warm climate kind of guy. That's me, permanent smile from ear to ear, all summer long. Sure, it's because I enjoy cycling and exercising outside and, yes, I love hanging out with the entire Wagman clan at the cottage on weekends, but my true love of summer is of course...food! From cherries and peaches to blueberries and corn, the summer yields so much flavorful locally grown produce I go wild!

In my part of the word, the beautiful robust strawberries that begin to appear at the markets are one of the first signs that summer is well and truly here. Unlike their impostor cousins (out-of-season strawberries that are imported from elsewhere), these berries are sweet with a strong nose — a term you might have heard someone use when describing the aroma, or bouquet, of a fine wine. I think it also works for fruit. As I've mentioned, I can be found smelling fruits and vegetables, fish and even meats while I'm shopping. In the absence of taste, the next best barometer is the nose of foods, literally their smell. In most cases the "nose knows" best.

My Mom's Applesauce

In every kitchen I have ever worked in, I have made this recipe. It goes with everything, from pork baby back ribs for a staff meal to foie gras served as an appetizer. It's really that good!

Makes about 3 cups (750 mL)

■ ■ ■

Chef Jordan's Tips

If you have leftover figs, dates or even bananas and plums, this recipe is a great opportunity to use them up. Simply substitute an equal quantity for the nectarines.

I prefer to use a food mill when making applesauce because it breaks down the skins, creating a wonderful texture that is difficult to achieve using a food processor.

Nutrition Tip

The pectin in apples helps keep your baby's bowels working well and is beneficial for her blood sugar level. They are also chock-full of immune-boosting vitamin C. Make sure you wash them well and leave the skins on, because the anti-inflammatory compound quercetin is found only in the apple skin.

Buy organic apples

7 cups	chopped cored McIntosh apples	1.75 L
2	nectarines, pitted	2
1/2 cup	freshly squeezed grapefruit juice	125 mL
1/2 cup	raw cane or granulated sugar	125 mL
1	stick cinnamon (2 inches/5 cm)	1

1. In a saucepan, combine apples, nectarines, grapefruit juice, sugar and cinnamon. Bring to a boil over medium-low heat. Reduce heat to low and simmer, stirring occasionally, until apples are soft, about 1 1/2 hours. Discard cinnamon stick.

2. Transfer to a food mill (see Tips, left) or food processor and process to desired consistency. Let cool to room temperature before serving or transfer to an airtight container and refrigerate for up to 3 days or freeze up to 6 months.

Nutrients per serving (1/2 cup/125 mL)

Calories 185	Dietary fiber . . . . . . 3.9 g
Protein . . . . 1.0 g	Sodium . . . . 19.8 mg
Total fat . . . . 1.4 g	Calcium . . . . 13.3 mg
Saturated fat. . . . . . 0.2 g	Iron . . . . 1.4 mg
Carbohydrates. . . . 43.9 g	Vitamin C. . . . . . . 8.9 mg

Not just for babies

If the recipe is left chunky, it becomes a wonderful chutney that you can serve with a pork tenderloin.

Frozen Mango Mousse

A cross between sorbet and granita (a granular Italian frozen ice dessert), this delicious dessert is good for you, too.

Makes about 2 cups (500 mL)

■ ■ ■

Chef Jordan's Tips

We recommend the use of pasteurized egg whites rather than raw egg whites because of the possibility of salmonella.

Since this recipe contains honey, be sure not to serve it to babies under 12 months of age.

Nutrition Tip

Along with its tropical cousins papayas and pineapples, mangoes contain a group of enzymes that help digestion. Some of these are called proteolytic enzymes, which means they break down proteins. The presence of these powerful enzymes explains why mangoes are often in meat tenderizers in the countries where they grow.

¼ cup	pasteurized egg whites (see Tips, left)	50 mL
1 tsp	granulated sugar	5 mL
1¾ cups	Mango Purée (see recipe, page 39)	425 mL
1 tsp	liquid honey	5 mL

1. In a bowl, whisk together egg whites and sugar vigorously to form stiff peaks. In a freezer-safe bowl, combine mango purée and honey. Fold whites into mango mixture until well blended.

2. Freeze for at least 4 hours, removing 5 or 6 times and scraping the mixture with the tines of a fork to create little "pebbles." Serve or cover tightly and freeze for up to 1 month. Let stand at room temperature for about 10 minutes before serving.

Nutrients per serving (¼ cup/50 mL)

Calories 26	Dietary fiber . . . . . . 0.3 g
Protein . . . . 0.9 g	Sodium . . . . 14.8 mg
Total fat . . . . 0.1 g	Calcium . . . . 1.5 mg
Saturated fat. . . . . . 0.0 g	Iron . . . . 0.0 mg
Carbohydrates. . . . . 5.4 g	Vitamin C. . . . . . . 2.3 mg

Not just for babies

Bon appetit. This will satisfy your family's craving for ice cream...most of the time.

Chocolate Macaroons

I prefer my macaroons on the smallish side, almost one-biters. When a recipe is this easy, can you really justify eating store-bought macaroons?

Makes about 18 macaroons

■ ■ ■

Chef Jordan's Tips

When egg whites are whisked to "stiff peaks" this literally means to whip them until they resemble a mountain range, stiff, with zero movement.

Nutrition Tip

Mmm, chocolate. From a health perspective, the best choice is high-quality, plain dark chocolate. The more the chocolate is processed, the more its polyphenols are lost. These polyphenols are potent antioxidants that help the body's cells resist damage. Dark chocolate retains much more of this antioxidant capability than milk chocolate does, plus it generally contains less sugar and butterfat. To reap the health benefits of chocolate look for the first ingredient to be "cacao" or "cocoa" or for the chocolate bar to contain at least 70% cocoa solids.

- Preheat oven to 350°F (180°C)
- Nonstick baking sheets

2	egg whites	2
1 tsp	agave nectar	5 mL
1 tsp	granulated sugar	5 mL
1 cup	unsweetened shredded coconut	250 mL
½ cup	milk or semisweet chocolate chips	125 mL

1. In a bowl, whisk egg whites, agave nectar and sugar until stiff peaks form. Stir in coconut and chocolate chips. Drop batter by tablespoonfuls (15 mL) onto baking sheets, 2 inches (5 cm) apart.

2. Bake in preheated oven until golden brown, about 10 minutes. Transfer to a wire rack and cool to room temperature before serving. Store in an airtight container at room temperature for up to 5 days.

Nutrients per macaroon			
Calories	68	Dietary fiber	0.7 g
Protein	1.2 g	Sodium	12.4 mg
Total fat	4.8 g	Calcium	1.3 mg
Saturated fat	3.5 g	Iron	0.1 mg
Carbohydrates	5.7 g	Vitamin C	0.1 mg

Not just for babies
These yummy cookies should be enjoyed by the entire family.

Pomegranate and Kiwi Purée with Crème Fraîche

The velvety texture of this recipe resembles a mousse or pudding — either way it's a hit!

Makes about 1¾ cups (425 mL)

■ ■ ■

Chef Jordan's Tips

You can use prepared pomegranate juice in this recipe so long as it is unsweetened, or you can make your own by pressing the seeds of a fresh pomegranate through a mesh strainer. Discard the seeds and use the juicy pulp in this recipe.

I prefer to whip the cream at the last moment because it tends to deflate rather quickly.

Crème fraîche is available in specialty food shops. If you can't find it, substitute an equal amount of sour cream in this recipe.

Nutrition Tip

Move over oranges — here comes the kiwi. Ounce for ounce, the kiwi contains more vitamin C than oranges, which have been a traditional source of this nutrient.

½ cup	pomegranate juice (see Tips, left)	125 mL
1 cup	chopped peeled fresh kiwi	250 mL
½ cup	pure maple syrup	125 mL
½ cup	crème fraîche	125 mL
½ cup	whipping (35%) cream, whipped	125 mL

1. In a blender, combine pomegranate juice, kiwi and syrup and purée until smooth. Transfer to a fine mesh strainer set over a bowl and strain, allowing the juice to flow naturally. Fold crème fraîche and whipped cream into juice.

2. Transfer solids to a saucepan and bring to a boil over medium heat. Cook until mixture is reduced by three-quarters, about 5 minutes. Set aside to cool until warm to the touch. To serve, drizzle some of the reduction over top of the "mousse." Serve immediately.

Nutrients per serving (¼ cup/50 mL)

Calories 155	Dietary fiber . . . . . . 0.8 g
Protein . . . . 1.1 g	Sodium . . . . 14.3 mg
Total fat . . . . 6.4 g	Calcium . . . . 45.6 mg
Saturated fat. . . . . . 3.8 g	Iron . . . . 0.4 mg
Carbohydrates. . . . 23.6 g	Vitamin C. . . . . . 24.8 mg

Not just for babies

Turn this into an elegant parfait. In a champagne glass, alternate layers of the pomegranate mixture with additional whipped cream. Garnish with pomegranate seeds, crushed toasted nuts and thin strands of fresh mint.

Cheesecake Soufflé

My signature dessert! What can I say? It's awesome.

Makes 4 child-size servings

■ ■ ■

Chef Jordan's Tips

A coating of sugar and butter creates indentations that give the soufflé mixture something to cling to while "scaling" the walls of the ramekin. An important step, indeed.

Egg whites beat much more easily and faster at room temperature, resulting in great volume because the proteins in the whites expand much better when warmed. This results in "perfect peaks."

- Preheat oven to 350°F (180°C)
- Four ½ cup (125 mL) ramekins
- Rimmed baking sheet

½ tsp	unsalted butter, softened	2 mL
1½ tbsp	granulated sugar, divided	22 mL
6 oz	cream cheese, softened	175 g
¼ cup	agave nectar	50 mL
2	eggs, separated, at room temperature (see Tips, left)	2
¼ cup	all-purpose flour	50 mL

1. Using your hands, evenly coat the inside of the ramekins with butter and sprinkle with ½ tbsp (7 mL) of the sugar, ensuring the sugar is equally distributed among the ramekins and they are entirely coated (see Tips, left).

2. In a bowl, whisk together cream cheese, agave nectar and remaining 1 tbsp (15 mL) of the sugar until sugar is dissolved and mixture is creamy. Whisk in egg yolks, one at a time, until well blended; set aside.

3. In another bowl, using a clean whisk, whisk egg whites until stiff peaks form. Fold in flour just to combine. Be sure not to overmix the egg whites as they'll lose volume quite quickly. Pour half of the egg whites into the cream cheese mixture and fold to combine. Fold in remaining egg whites. Divide evenly between the prepared ramekins. Place ramekins on rimmed baking sheet and pour hot water into the bottom of the baking sheet, about ¼ of the way up the ramekin. Bake in preheated oven until the tops of the soufflés have puffed and are golden brown, about 30 minutes. Serve immediately to adults or let cool to luke warm and remove from the ramekins if you're serving children.

Not just for babies

If you like cheesecake, you should have the pleasure of eating a cheesecake soufflé. A presentation that will set you apart is to bring the individual soufflés to the table and poke a hole into the middle of each, creating a cavern to accept anything from melted chocolate to berry purées. Enjoy!

Nutrition Tip

Agave syrup or nectar is produced from the agave plant, which is native to Mexico. No chemicals are used in its extraction and the syrup is available in light (filtered) or dark (unfiltered) versions. Perhaps not surprisingly, the unfiltered retains more of its minerals, which include calcium, magnesium and iron. Agave nectar contains a high percentage of fructose, which makes it much sweeter than sucrose or honey. It can be used as a more healthful sweetener choice than regular sugar and is available in most natural food stores.

Maple Syrup-Glazed Pineapple

This is the "northern" way of eating pineapple, coated with maple syrup and served while it's snowing outside. But it's so good you can enjoy it any time of the year. Serve this to your toddler after her first birthday has passed.

Makes about 2 cups (500 mL)

▪ ▪ ▪

Chef Jordan's Tips

Feel free to grill the pineapple slices on the barbecue prior to dicing. This adds a wonderful smoky dimension to the dessert.

If time is your enemy, by all means purchase a pineapple that has been peeled and cored and stored in its own juices. I do, however, recommend that you open the storage container to verify its freshness. Remember, "the nose knows"!

Nutrition Tip

Not only does pure maple syrup taste wonderful, it also provides the minerals manganese and zinc. Manganese is important for diminishing the harmful effects of free radicals in the body's cells, and zinc provides a nice boost for the immune system.

- Potato masher, optional

2 tbsp	unsalted butter	25 mL
2½ cups	diced fresh pineapple	625 mL
1 tbsp	pure maple syrup	15 mL

1. In a saucepan, melt butter over medium heat. Add pineapple and cook, without stirring, until all liquid from pineapple has evaporated and the chunks begin to caramelize, about 8 minutes. Stir in syrup, reduce heat to low and cook until pineapple is fully coated, about 1 minute. Mash or cut to desired consistency. Let cool to room temperature or transfer to an airtight container and refrigerate for up to 3 days.

Nutrients per serving (¼ cup/50 mL)	
Calories 56	Dietary fiber . . . . . . 0.7 g
Protein . . . . 0.3 g	Sodium . . . . 1.1 mg
Total fat . . . . 2.9 g	Calcium . . . . 9.2 mg
Saturated fat. . . . . . 1.8 g	Iron . . . . 0.2 mg
Carbohydrates. . . . . 8.1 g	Vitamin C. . . . . . 18.5 mg

Not just for babies

I rarely use alcohol in my baking or desserts, but once in awhile a flavor combination is destined to be together. After scooping off enough to mash for Baby, Mom and Dad can add a splash of good rum and allow to cook for another 2 minutes while the alcohol is cooked out, leaving that tropical flavor typically reserved for the seaside in the Caribbean.

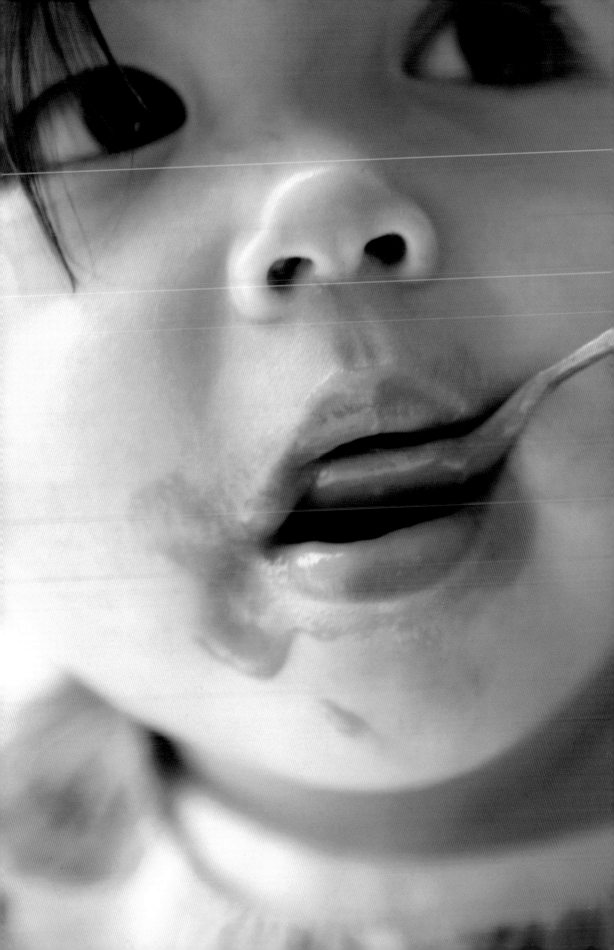

Pacific Salmon Cakes (page 155)

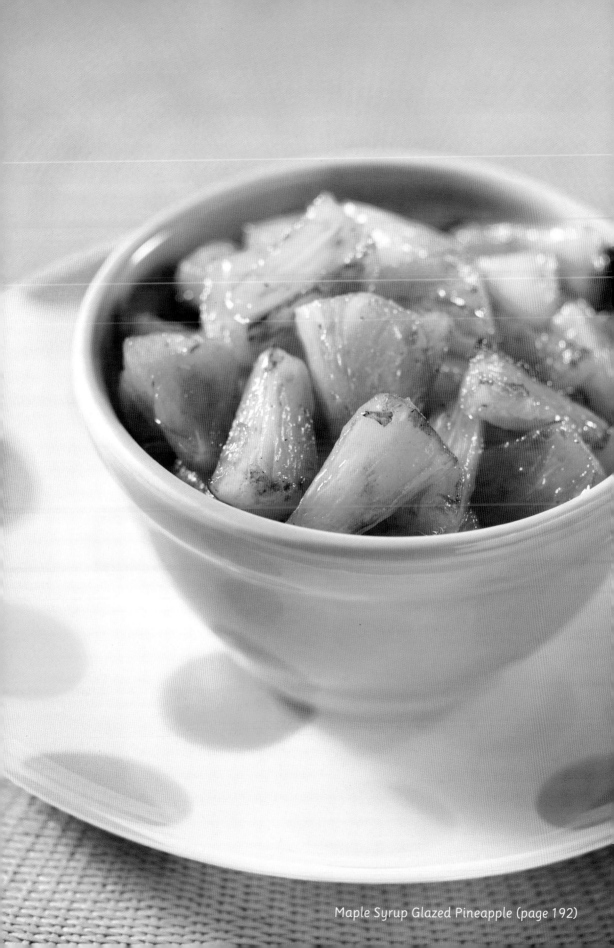

Maple Syrup Glazed Pineapple (page 192)

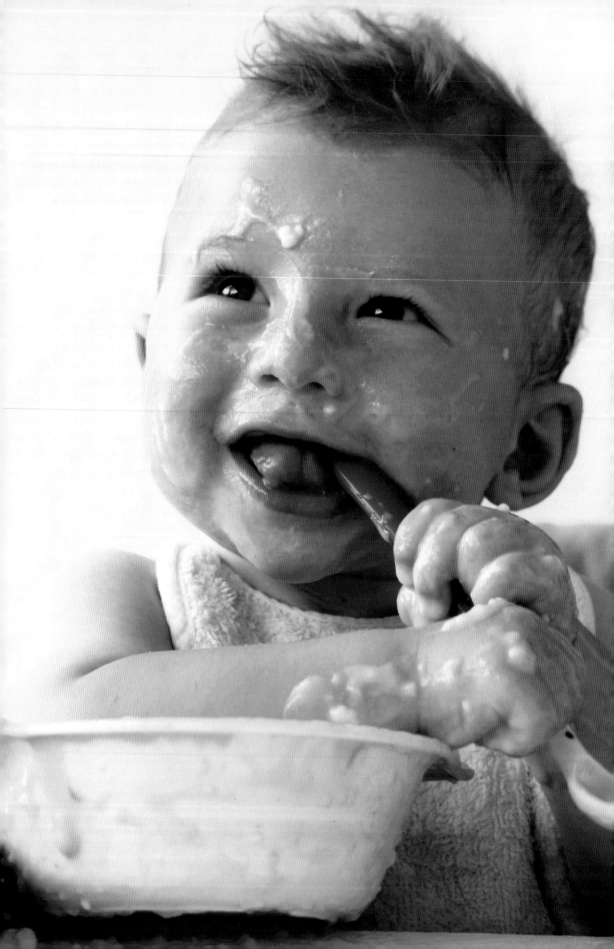

Short-Grain Brown Rice Pudding with Chocolate Wafers

A chocolate rice pudding! Seriously, where was this recipe when I was growing up?

Makes about 5 cups (1.25 L)

▪ ▪ ▪

Chef Jordan's Tips

Freshly shaved chocolate is a tasty garnish for this pudding. Use dark, milk or even white chocolate — all will taste great!

Nutrition Tip

Brown rice is a good source of the trace mineral selenium, an antioxidant that many North Americans do not get enough of in their diet. Accumulating evidence suggests a strong inverse relationship between selenium and the incidence of cancer.

For an added nutritional kick, substitute dried cranberries and dark chocolate chunks for the chocolate wafer cookies.

1 tbsp	unsalted butter	15 mL
1½ cups	short-grain brown rice, rinsed	375 mL
5 cups	whole milk	1.25 L
¼ cup	agave nectar	50 mL
¾ cup	pure maple syrup	175 mL
1½ cups	crushed chocolate wafer cookies	375 mL

1. In a saucepan, melt butter over medium-low heat. Stir in rice, mixing to thoroughly coat grains. Add milk, agave nectar and maple syrup and bring to a boil. Reduce heat to low and simmer, stirring occasionally, until liquid begins to thicken, about 10 minutes. Cover, remove from heat and set aside to finish cooking, about 2 hours.

2. Stir in chocolate wafer cookies. Serve warm or cold.

Nutrients per serving (¼ cup/50 mL)	
Calories 180	Dietary fiber . . . . . . 0.9 g
Protein . . . . 3.8 g	Sodium . . . . 77.0 mg
Total fat . . . . 4.2 g	Calcium . . . . 86.1 mg
Saturated fat. . . . . . 1.9 g	Iron . . . . 0.7 mg
Carbohydrates. . . . 32.4 g	Vitamin C. . . . . . . 0.0 mg

Not just for babies

If you have leftovers, divide cold pudding into 1 tbsp (15 mL) portions and roll in panko bread crumbs. Freeze, if desired. When you're ready to serve, preheat 4 cups (1 L) canola oil to 300°F (150°C). Fry, in batches, until golden brown, about 3 minutes. Rest on paper towel to absorb excess oil. Serve warm.

Berry-Glazed Fig Tart

A traditional French classic made easy for you! Since this tart contains sliced fruit, we recommend serving it to babies who have passed their first birthday.

Makes about 8 servings

■ ■ ■

Chef Jordan's Tips

Egg wash, which can be either straight beaten egg yolk or egg yolk mixed with a bit of water has many uses, from "fastening" pieces of puff pastry to encouraging a golden brown finish on pies.

Nutrition Tip

The combination of blueberries, apples and figs in this recipe makes it very tasty and a very good source of dietary fiber. Eating enough fiber not only helps balance blood sugar and cholesterol levels but also helps the colon rid the body of toxins.

Buy organic apples

- Preheat oven to 300°F (150°C)
- Baking sheet

Glaze

¾ cup	blueberries	175 mL
¼ cup	water	50 mL
1 tbsp	agave nectar	15 mL
1 tbsp	raspberry preserves	15 mL

Tart

2 tbsp	all-purpose flour	25 mL
½	package (1 lb/500 g) frozen puff pastry, thawed	½
1	egg, beaten	1
1 cup	sliced cored peeled apples	250 mL
1 cup	fresh figs, halved	250 mL
1 tbsp	packed brown sugar	15 mL
1 tsp	grated lemon zest	5 mL

1. *Glaze:* In a saucepan, combine blueberries, water, agave nectar and raspberry preserves. Bring to a boil over medium heat and cook until liquid is reduced by about three-quarters, about 6 minutes. Let cool to room temperature.

2. *Tart:* On a lightly floured surface, roll out pastry into a 10-inch (25 cm) square. Trim a ½-inch (1 cm) strip from all four sides; set strips aside. Place pastry on a baking sheet and brush edges with egg. Place the four strips back on the edges of larger piece (the egg will "glue" the strips into place), trimming the excess.

3. In a bowl, combine apples, figs, brown sugar and lemon zest.

4. To assemble the tart, pour the glaze onto the puff pastry and distribute evenly, keeping it inside the raised edge. Spoon the apple mixture onto the glaze and spread out to distribute evenly. Bake in preheated oven until pastry is golden brown and bottom is cooked, about 30 minutes. Let cool on the baking sheet to room temperature before serving.

Nutrients per serving	
Calories 329	Dietary fiber . . . . . . 2.2 g
Protein . . . . 5.9 g	Sodium . . . . . . 313.7 mg
Total fat . . . . 17.5 g	Calcium . . . . 5.8 mg
Saturated fat. . . . . . 4.8 g	Iron . . . . 2.0 mg
Carbohydrates. . . . 37.4 g	Vitamin C. . . . . . . 5.6 mg

Not just for babies
This delicate tart is light enough to be served with afternoon tea or as a dessert at lunch, as well as after dinner.

Cranberry Phyllo "Pinwheels"

A simple and elegant (and don't forget almost healthy) way to introduce your children to the world of tart, but nutritious, cranberries. It will be also a welcome addition to your holiday repertoire.

Makes about 10 servings

■ ■ ■

Chef Jordan's Tips

When cooked, the butter and phyllo dough layers create distinct crispy layers of goodness similar to puff pastry. However, phyllo dough is made without butter, unlike puff pastry. That's why it's imperative to alternate layers of dough and butter.

Frozen cranberries will substitute well for fresh but I would not recommend using canned cranberries for this recipe because they often contain a tremendous amount of added sugar.

- Preheat oven to 300°F (150°C)
- Baking sheet

3 cups	fresh cranberries	750 mL
½ cup	agave nectar	125 mL
½ cup	pure maple syrup	125 mL
1 tbsp	grated lemon zest	15 mL
¼ cup	quick-cooking oats	50 mL
4	sheets phyllo pastry (each 10-inches/25 cm square)	4
¼ cup	unsalted butter, melted	50 mL
1 cup	full-fat sour cream	250 mL
¼ cup	icing sugar, sifted	50 mL

1. In a saucepan, combine cranberries, agave nectar and maple syrup and lemon zest. Bring to a boil over medium heat. Reduce heat to low and simmer, stirring occasionally, until berries are soft and "splitting" open, about 30 minutes. Remove from heat and stir in oats. Let cool to room temperature.

2. On a cutting board, working with 1 sheet at a time, brush phyllo with melted butter (see Tips, left), stacking sheets as completed to create 4 layers. Spread cranberry mixture over the surface leaving about a 1-inch (2.5 cm) border around the edges. Starting at one edge roll pastry tightly and continue rolling until finished. It should resemble a jelly roll. Place on baking sheet. Bake in preheated oven until golden brown, about 30 minutes. Let cool to room temperature on baking sheet on a wire rack.

3. In a bowl, whisk together sour cream and icing sugar. To serve, spread the "icing" over the bottom of a serving dish. Cut rolls into 1½-inch thick (4 cm) slices and place "pinwheel" on top of icing.

Nutrients per serving	
Calories 200	Dietary fiber . . . . . . 1.5 g
Protein . . . . 1.1 g	Sodium . . . . 10.1 mg
Total fat . . . . 7.9 g	Calcium . . . . 29.3 mg
Saturated fat. . . . . . 5.2 g	Iron . . . . 0.2 mg
Carbohydrates. . . . 30.8 g	Vitamin C. . . . . . . 4.6 mg

Not just for babies

Everyone in the family can enjoy this as is. For a more sophisticated presentation, pass the unglazed pinwheels with a bowl of the "icing" and allow guests to dip. Pass lots of napkins, too.

Nutrition Tip

Cranberries have long been valued as a treatment for urinary tract infections, but new research from the University of Rochester shows they may be able to help prevent cavities, too. Two flavonoids in cranberries, quercetin and myricetin, have been found to reduce plaque formation on teeth, stop bacteria from sticking to the teeth and reduce the acid conditions that can start the decay process. The cranberry season is short, so when they are available, make sure you freeze some to have on hand throughout the year.

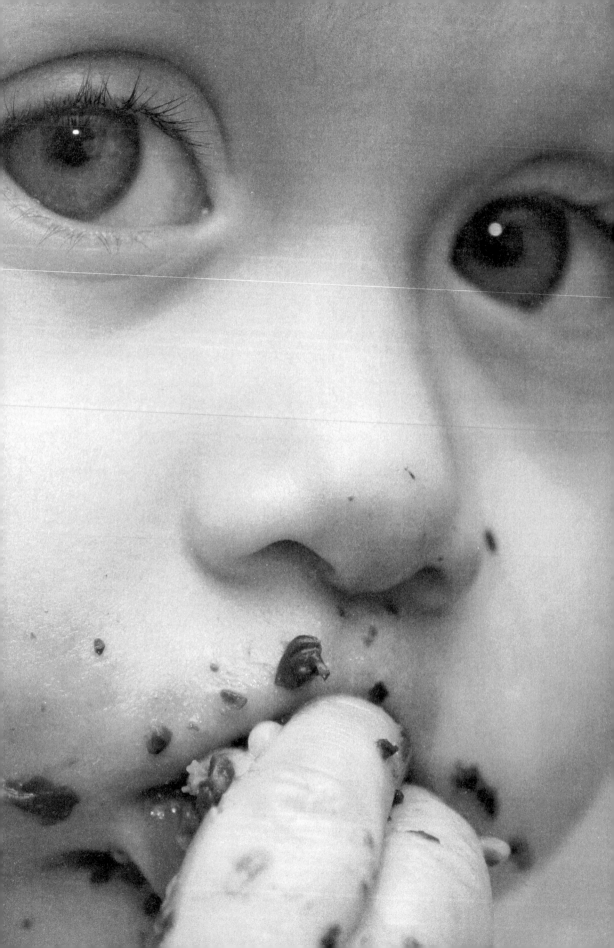

Not for Adults Only

Introduction 200

Vegetable Stock 201
Roasted Chicken Stock 202
Roasted Cherry Tomato
    Vinaigrette 204
Roasted Red Pepper
    Vinaigrette 205
Lemon Horseradish Aioli 206
Caper and Lemon Remoulade 207
Oven-Roasted Red Peppers 208
Basic Sweet-and-Sour Sauce 209
Cucumber Salad with
    Smoked Salmon 210
Chickpea, Grape Tomato
    and Feta Salad 212
Roasted Beet Salad 214
Barley Salad with Apples and
    Sugar Snap Peas 215
Poached Whole Artichokes
    with Lemon Horseradish Aioli . . . 216
Honey Mustard-Glazed Salmon
    with Avocado 218

Grilled Portobello Mushroom
    Stack with Goat Cheese 220
Poppy Seed-Crusted Yellowfin
    Tuna with Roasted Shallots 222
Israeli Couscous with Black Tiger
    Shrimp and Shrimp "Bisque" . . . 224
Butter-Crusted Black Cod
    with Heirloom Tomatoes 226
Salmon en Croute with
    Arugula Salad 228
Whole Roasted Chicken Stuffed
    with Lime and Green Onions 230
Citrus BBQ-Glazed Baby
    Back Ribs 232
Oven-Roasted Cornish Hen
    with Sage 234
"Cassoulet" of Black-Eyed Peas,
    Chorizo Sausage and NY Steak . . 236
Veal Rib Chops with Fresh Corn
    and Asparagus Succotash 238
Sliced NY Steak with Mushroom
    Duxelles and Fresh Horseradish . . 240
Spice-Rubbed Rack of Lamb 242

Introduction

Although the recipes in this chapter are primarily for adults, given our philosophy of eating, we recommend sharing portions with your toddler in appropriately sized bites or, depending on your baby's stage of development, combining a small portion of the recipe with a vegetable purée. We've included suggested combinations in the Just for babies feature accompanying each recipe.

We strongly believe in sharing a wide range of foods with your children from their earliest days. Feeding your children different tastes and textures helps them develop a well-rounded palate and a healthy sense of adventure about trying new and interesting foods. This makes meal preparation easier not only because you won't have to prepare separate "child only" dishes for picky eaters, but also because exposing your children to a wide variety of foods encourages them to develop healthy eating habits that will serve them well throughout their lifetimes. Eating a varied diet is one of the single best ways to ensure they get the full range of nutrients they need to enjoy optimal health at every stage of their lives. Preparing a delicious dinner for yourselves and sharing it with your children is also an opportunity to enjoy the kind of quality family time that is associated with mental well-being, as well as physical health.

We have also included some basic recipes, such as vegetable and chicken stock and roasted red peppers, that you can use when preparing dishes for your baby that call for these items.

Vegetable Stock

I like to use this as a cooking liquid instead of water in many dishes because it adds flavor. It doesn't contain any preservatives or added salt, as do prepared stocks.

Makes about 8 cups (2 L)

■ ■ ■

Chef Jordan's Tips

When making stock be sure not to overboil it. After 45 minutes all the flavor will have been leached from the vegetables and continuing to cook will not enhance it.

Nutrition Tip

Other than its superior taste, the major benefits of homemade stock are that you can control the amount of salt and you know what it contains. A serving-size portion of a commercial brand can provide up to one-third the recommended daily intake of sodium for adults. Commercial products may also contain other flavor enhancers, such as monosodium glutamate (MSG), which may not be noted on the label. MSG is listed only if it appears in its pure form, not if it is part of another ingredient such as hydrolyzed vegetable protein.

- Large stock pot
- Fine mesh strainer

10 cups	water	2.5 L
2 cups	coarsely chopped peeled carrots	500 mL
2 cups	chopped onions	500 mL
1 cup	coarsely chopped celery	250 mL
1 cup	coarsely chopped parsnip	250 mL
1 cup	garlic cloves	250 mL

1. In stock pot, combine water, carrots, onions, celery, parsnips and garlic. Bring to a boil over medium heat. Reduce heat to low and simmer until broth is flavorful, about 45 minutes. In a fine mesh strainer set over a pot or bowl, strain out solids and discard. Cover and refrigerate for up to 3 days or freeze in airtight containers for up to 3 months.

Nutrients per serving (1 cup/250 mL)	
Calories 72	Dietary fiber . . . . . . 3.1 g
Protein . . . . 2.2 g	Sodium . . . . 51.2 mg
Total fat . . . . 0.3 g	Calcium . . . . 73.2 mg
Saturated fat . . . . . . 0.1 g	Iron . . . . 0.6 mg
Carbohydrates . . . . 16.4 g	Vitamin C . . . . . . 13.9 mg

Just for babies

Use this stock in place of water to cook vegetables, for purées once all the ingredients it contains have been introduced to your child, or to thin them if you're freezing in ice cube trays. You can also use it instead of water to cook grains such as rice, barley, millet or quinoa for added flavor.

Roasted Chicken Stock

This is the mother of all stocks. It can be used to enhance the flavor of just about everything from rice and barley to poached chicken and beef.

Makes about 14 cups (3.5 L)

■ ■ ■

Chef Jordan's Tips

Try shredding the cooked chicken and using it in tacos.

Nutrition Tip

Rich chicken stock has always been a valued remedy for the flu, and for good reason. In order to fight infection, the body needs many resources, including the easily absorbable minerals from the bones, marrow and cartilage that go into a good broth. Fish bones and heads can also be used in the same way to make a fish stock high in iodine, a mineral in short supply in North American diets.

- Preheat oven to 450°F (230°C)
- Large ovenproof skillet
- Large stock pot
- Fine mesh strainer

1 tbsp	extra virgin olive oil	15 mL
1	whole chicken, cut into quarters (about 3 lbs/1.5 kg)	1
16 cups	water	4 L
2 cups	chopped celery	500 mL
2 cups	chopped peeled parsnips	500 mL
1½ cups	chopped peeled carrots	375 mL
1½ cups	chopped onions	375 mL
6	cloves garlic	6
½ cup	fresh parsley sprigs	125 mL
1 tsp	whole black peppercorns	5 mL
2	bay leaves	2

1. In ovenproof skillet, heat oil over medium heat. Add chicken pieces, skin side down, and transfer skillet to preheated oven. Roast until chicken is golden brown, about 35 minutes.

2. Transfer chicken to the stock pot, being sure to add all the bits from the bottom of the skillet.

3. Add water, celery, parsnips, carrots, onions, garlic, parsley, peppercorns and bay leaves to the pot. Bring to a boil over high heat. Reduce heat to low and simmer, skimming the impurities that rise to the surface, until liquid is flavorful and chicken is fully cooked, about 40 minutes.

4. In a fine mesh strainer set over a bowl or clean pot, strain the stock, reserving the chicken for another use and discarding vegetables. Let the stock cool to room temperature. Transfer to airtight containers and refrigerate for up to 3 days or freeze for up to 3 months.

Nutrients per serving (1 cup/250 mL)	
Calories 254	Dietary fiber . . . . . . 2.1 g
Protein . . . . 17.5 g	Sodium . . . . . . 102.9 mg
Total fat . . . . 16.6 g	Calcium . . . . 47.8 mg
Saturated fat . . . . . . 4.6 g	Iron . . . . 1.4 mg
Carbohydrates . . . . . 8.0 g	Vitamin C . . . . 9.6 mg

Just for babies

There are many recipes in this book to which the addition of roasted chicken stock will contribute added depth of flavor. For instance, use it to replace the water in Bok Choy with Fresh Ginger (see recipe, page 92) or Brussels Sprouts with Bacon (see recipe, page 93). If it's available, stock is usually preferable to water in most recipes.

Roasted Cherry Tomato Vinaigrette

This vinaigrette is a staple in the Wagman fridge. We use it on everything from salads to grilled asparagus.

Makes about 2½ cups (625 mL)

■ ■ ■

Chef Jordan's Tips
Champagne, cider and sherry are among my favorite vinegars, but pear is at the top of the list. In this recipe, it contrasts beautifully with the tomato.

Nutrition Tip
Tomatoes contain more lycopene than any other fruit or vegetable. This red carotenoid has received a lot of attention specifically for its potential to reduce the risk of prostate cancer. In one study, Harvard researchers found that men who ate more than two ½-cup (125 mL) servings of tomato sauce every week were 23 per cent less likely to develop prostate cancer during the duration of the study (22 years) than the men who ate less than one serving of tomato sauce per month.

1½ cups	Oven-Roasted Cherry Tomato Purée (see recipe, page 94)	375 mL
½ cup	extra virgin olive oil	125 mL
½ cup	sherry, balsamic or pear vinegar (see Tips, left)	125 mL
3	cloves garlic, minced	3
1 tsp	kosher salt	5 mL
1 tsp	freshly ground black pepper	5 mL

1. In a bowl, whisk together cherry tomato purée, oil, vinegar, garlic, salt and pepper. The vinaigrette will be separated and not emulsified, so be sure to whisk it well immediately before using. Transfer to an airtight container and store in the refrigerator for up to 1 month.

Nutrients per ¼ cup (50 mL)

Calories 111	Dietary fiber . . . . . . 0.5 g
Protein . . . . 0.4 g	Sodium . . . . . . 585.8 mg
Total fat . . . . 11.5 g	Calcium . . . . 6.9 mg
Saturated fat. . . . . . 1.6 g	Iron . . . . 0.2 mg
Carbohydrates. . . . . 1.7 g	Vitamin C. . . . . . . 3.6 mg

Just for babies
This very versatile vinaigrette is delicate and mild enough that your older baby (9 to 12 months) can enjoy it, too. It would be a perfect dressing for steamed asparagus or added to plain yogurt as a dip for pita or soft vegetables.

Roasted Red Pepper Vinaigrette

Here's another vinaigrette we enjoy regularly in the Wagman home. Our son, Jonah, loves it, but growing up in our home, he's developed a discerning palate.

**Makes about
2¼ cups (550 mL)**

■ ■ ■

Chef Jordan's Tips

If you don't have sherry vinegar, rice or champagne vinegar also works well in this recipe.

My favorite sandwich is leftover meatloaf saturated with this vinaigrette and served between challah or egg bread. Virtually any leftover meat, sliced thin, including Thanksgiving turkey, would be excellent.

Nutrition Tip

Bell peppers can be a delicious tool to help keep your heart healthy. Among other beneficial compounds, peppers contain vitamin C, flavonoids and capsaicin. All three have been shown to decrease blood clot formation and reduce the risk of heart attack and stroke.

Buy organic peppers

1 cup	Oven-Roasted Red Peppers, puréed (see recipe, page 208)	250 mL
½ cup	extra virgin olive oil	125 mL
¼ cup	sherry vinegar (see Tips, left)	50 mL
1 tbsp	liquid honey	15 mL
2 tsp	kosher salt	10 mL
2 tsp	freshly ground black pepper	10 mL

1. In a bowl, whisk together roasted red pepper purée, oil, vinegar, honey, salt and pepper. The vinaigrette will be somewhat separated, so be sure to whisk it well immediately before using. Transfer to an airtight container and store in the refrigerator for up to 1 month.

Nutrients per ¼ cup (50 mL)	
Calories 132	Dietary fiber . . . . . . 0.4 g
Protein . . . . 0.2 g	Sodium . . . . . . 649.6 mg
Total fat . . . . 13.4 g	Calcium . . . . 3.2 mg
Saturated fat. . . . . . 1.9 g	Iron . . . . 0.1 mg
Carbohydrates. . . . . 2.9 g	Vitamin C. . . . . . 11.0 mg

Just for babies

If your baby is old enough to tolerate peppers (9 months +) try adding this to plain yogurt and serving it as a dip for soft vegetables or pita. A tiny amount would also enhance the flavor of Roasted Beet Purée (see recipe, page 46) or Diced Potato Gratin (see recipe, page 87).

Lemon Horseradish Aioli

This all-purpose sauce is great with everything from artichokes to fish.

Makes about ¼ cup (50 mL)

■ ■ ■

Nutrition Tip

Horseradish is a cruciferous vegetable that offers some protection against food-borne illness. It is estimated that there are 76 million cases of food-borne illness every year in the United States. Scientific investigation shows that horseradish can help protect against listeria, *E. coli* and *Staphylococcus aureus*, all of which cause typical food poisoning symptoms and can be very serious, especially for the very young, the very old and those with compromised immune systems. The chemical responsible for this protection, allyl isothiocyanate, is formed when the fresh horseradish is cut or chopped. However, this doesn't mean that you can be less diligent with hygiene. If you have any concerns or suspect food poisoning, see your doctor immediately.

2 tbsp	mayonnaise	25 mL
1 tbsp	freshly grated horseradish (or strained prepared horseradish)	15 mL
1 tsp	capers, rinsed thoroughly (see Tips, page 207)	5 mL
1 tsp	finely grated lemon zest	5 mL
1 tbsp	freshly squeezed lemon juice	15 mL
Pinch	freshly ground black pepper	Pinch
Pinch	salt, preferably kosher	Pinch

1. In a bowl, combine mayonnaise, horseradish, capers, lemon zest and juice, pepper and salt. Cover and refrigerate overnight or for up to 3 days.

Nutrients per 2 tbsp (25 mL)

Calories 109	Dietary fiber . . . . . . 0.2 g
Protein. . . . . 0.3 mg	Sodium . . . . . . 332.2 mg
Total fat. . . . . . . 11.2 mg	Calcium . . . . 10.9 mg
Saturated fat . . . . 1.5 mg	Iron . . . . 0.1 mg
Carbohydrates. . . . . 2.0 g	Vitamin C. . . . . . 13.5 mg

Just for babies

Try a dollop of this on Fennel and Apple-Stuffed Pork Chops (see recipe, page 158) or Red Cabbage with Duck Confit (see recipe, page 167) or add a bit to any meat to moisten and add flavor.

Caper and Lemon Remoulade

A wonderful accompaniment to any fish!

Makes about ½ cup (125 mL)

■ ■ ■

Chef Jordan's Tips

Capers are packed in brine and as a result can be very salty and quite tart. When introducing your children to capers, rinse them thoroughly under cold running water to wash away the briny flavor.

Nutrition Tip

Limonoids are compounds found in lemons that have been shown to help fight certain cancers, including skin, lung, breast and colon cancer. One of the things that makes this compound so potent is that it is very easily absorbed and utilized by the body (bioavailable). It also stays in the body, exerting positive effects for up to 24 hours.

Because you are using the zest of the lemon in this recipe, make sure it's organic.

½ cup	mayonnaise (see Tips, page 216)	125 mL
1 tsp	capers, rinsed, drained and minced (see Tips, left)	5 mL
1 tsp	grated lemon zest	5 mL
1 tsp	freshly squeezed lemon juice	5 mL

1. In a bowl, combine mayonnaise, capers, lemon zest and juice. Serve immediately or cover and refrigerate for up to 1 week.

Nutrients per ½ cup (125mL)	
Calories 848	Dietary fiber . . . . . . 0.2 g
Protein . . . . 0.3 g	Sodium . . . . . . 950.9 mg
Total fat. . . . . 93 g	Calcium . . . . 4.9 mg
Saturated fat. . . . . . 8.5 g	Iron . . . . 0.1 mg
Carbohydrates. . . . . 0.9 g	Vitamin C. . . . . . . 5.0 mg

Just for babies

Well, not really. The whole family can enjoy this with World's Best "Fish Sticks" (see recipe, page 150).

Oven-Roasted Red Peppers

This recipe is a staple in my home because it is so versatile.

Makes 12 servings

■ ■ ■

Chef Jordan's Tips

If time is not of the essence, allow the peppers to cool overnight in the refrigerator before peeling, which makes them easier to peel.

Use orange, red or yellow peppers for roasting because they tend to be the sweetest.

Nutrition Tip

Sweet red peppers are actually green peppers that have been allowed to ripen on the vine. Because of this ripening process they have significantly higher levels of nutrients and phytochemicals than green peppers. Select peppers that are firm, heavy for their size and without wrinkles to ensure you are getting those that are freshest and therefore most nutritious.

Buy organic peppers

- Preheat oven to 350°F (180°C)
- Large ovenproof skillet

6	red bell peppers	6
1 tbsp	extra virgin olive oil	15 mL
2	sprigs fresh thyme	2
2 tbsp	finely chopped basil leaves, divided	25 mL
Pinch	kosher salt	Pinch
Pinch	freshly ground black pepper	Pinch

1. In large ovenproof skillet, combine red peppers, oil, thyme, 1 tbsp (15 mL) of the basil, salt and pepper. Toss to thoroughly coat. Roast in preheated oven, turning peppers every 10 minutes, until all sides are golden brown and soft, about 1 hour. Let cool to room temperature (see Tips, left).

2. Set a fine mesh strainer over a bowl. Holding peppers over the strainer, remove skins, stems and seeds while catching all residual cooking liquid in the mixing bowl. Combine the peeled peppers, reserved liquid and remaining basil. Mix well.

Nutrients per ½ pepper	
Calories 26	Dietary fiber . . . . . . 1.2 g
Protein . . . . 0.6 g	Sodium . . . . 2.4 mg
Total fat . . . . 1.4 g	Calcium . . . . 4.9 mg
Saturated fat. . . . . . 0.2 g	Iron . . . . 0.3 mg
Carbohydrates. . . . . 3.6 g	Vitamin C. . . . . . 76.1 mg

Just for babies

Chop roasted peppers and combine with cooked noodles to create an excellent pasta dish for your baby (9 months +).

Basic Sweet-and-Sour Sauce

This will become a staple in your home, too...the all-purpose dip and spread! Try this sauce with fish sticks or chicken fingers for the kids or with a pork chop or salmon for Mom and Dad.

**Makes about
¾ cup (175 mL)**

■ ■ ■

Nutrition Tip

Sweet-and-sour sauce is a mainstay in Asian cooking and a favorite of many North Americans. But commercial sauces can be full of additives that may cause real problems for some people. Some sauces can have very high levels of sugar and salt, not to mention additives such as food coloring and monosodium glutamate, or MSG.

¼ cup	finely diced sweet onion	50 mL
¼ cup	extra virgin olive oil	50 mL
2 tbsp	rice vinegar	25 mL
2 tbsp	liquid honey	25 mL
2 tbsp	tamari (soy) sauce	25 mL
1 tbsp	grated peeled parsnip	15 mL
1 tbsp	grated peeled carrot	15 mL
1 tbsp	freshly squeezed lemon juice	15 mL
2	cloves garlic, minced	2
1 tsp	toasted sesame oil	5 mL

1. In a bowl, combine onion, oil, vinegar, honey, tamari, parsnip, carrot, lemon juice, garlic and sesame oil. Cover and refrigerate overnight or for up to 3 days.

Nutrients per ¼ cup (50 mL)	
Calories 200	Dietary fiber ...... 0.5 g
Protein .... 0.3 g	Sodium .... 2.7 mg
Total fat .... 15.8 g	Calcium .... 8.4 mg
Saturated fat...... 2.2 g	Iron .... 0.1 mg
Carbohydrates.... 14.4 g	Vitamin C....... 4.5 mg

Just for babies

Since this sauce contains honey, don't serve it to babies younger than 1 year. For a change serve this with World's Best "Fish Sticks" (see recipe, page 150), instead of the remoulade.

Cucumber Salad with Smoked Salmon

This recipe is awesome! It reminds me of warm summer days, sitting on the porch of my family's summer home looking out at the lake. It doesn't get better than that.

Makes 2 servings

■ ■ ■

Chef Jordan's Tips

I've always said people begin to learn the most when they confess to knowing very little. As chef of Pascal in Newport Beach, Calif., I was fortunate to work with a man by the name of Procoro, who was the self-proclaimed king of cold salads. I learned so much from him, from salting the cucumber for the salad to develop the texture to bringing champagne vinegar to a boil with tarragon to create a quick infusion for a vinaigrette. We all keep learning — that's the best part about cuisine and life in general.

2 cups	coarsely chopped seeded peeled English cucumber	500 mL
1 tsp	kosher salt	5 mL
1 cup	corn kernels, cooked	250 mL
¾ cup	finely chopped peeled celery	175 mL
⅓ cup	full-fat yogurt	75 mL
2 tbsp	white wine vinegar	25 mL
1 tsp	finely chopped fresh dill	5 mL
½ tsp	freshly ground black pepper	2 mL
6	smoked salmon slices (about 6 oz/175 g)	6
1 tbsp	chopped chives	15 mL

1. In a bowl, combine cucumber and salt; set aside for at least 30 minutes or for up to 1 hour to soften the cucumber. Drain off liquid leached from cucumber and add corn, celery, yogurt, vinegar, dill and pepper, stirring to coat evenly. Cover and refrigerate overnight.

2. To serve, cover the bottom of each plate with a few pieces of smoked salmon. Using a slotted spoon, place salad on top of salmon. Drizzle some of the vinaigrette around salmon and garnish with chopped chives. Serve immediately.

Nutrients per serving			
Calories	241	Dietary fiber	6.0 g
Protein	21.7 g	Sodium	825.7 mg
Total fat	6.5 g	Calcium	155.9 mg
Saturated fat	1.9 g	Iron	1.9 mg
Carbohydrates	26.2 g	Vitamin C	16.9 mg

Just for babies

The entire family can enjoy this salad together...just make sure you dice the salmon in the baby's portion. My son, Jonah, has always enjoyed smoked salmon, whether in his scrambled eggs in the morning or over a Crispy Potato Galette (see recipe, page 132). I guarantee your kids will love it, too! This is a great dish to serve when the grandparents come for brunch.

Nutrition Tip

Salmon is an excellent source of beautiful polyunsaturated omega-3 fatty acids. But how do farmed salmon compare to wild? The United States Department of Agriculture (USDA) states that wild salmon have a 20 per cent higher protein content but 20 per cent less fat than farmed. Both types still offer beneficial levels of omega-3 fats, but the farmed fish have higher levels of omega-6 fatty acids (because they are grain fed). Studies suggest the ratio of omega-6 to omega-3 fats in our diets is between 10:1 and 20:1, which is too high in omega-6. Omega-6 fatty acids break down into inflammatory compounds in the body, and their excessive consumption is associated with conditions such as heart disease, diabetes and arthritis.

Chickpea, Grape Tomato and Feta Salad

This hearty and very fresh-tasting salad makes a great lunch all on its own. And it gets even better as it sits in your refrigerator. The trouble is, it never lasts very long.

Makes 6 to 8 servings

■ ■ ■

Chef Jordan's Tips

Peeled celery? I've found that more often than not, celery gets a bad rap in my house. One of the tricks for using celery, either cooked or raw, is to peel the fibrous side using a regular vegetable peeler. As you peel you'll see the "strands" of celery being peeled away exposing a fleshy white vegetable. That's exactly what you want.

- Preheat oven to 300°F (150°C)

Vinaigrette

1 tbsp	grated lemon zest	15 mL
¼ cup	freshly squeezed lemon juice	50 mL
2 tbsp	extra virgin olive oil	25 mL
1 tbsp	minced garlic	15 mL

Salad

2½ lbs	grape tomatoes	1.25 kg
6 cups	drained canned or cooked chickpeas (see page 77)	1.5 L
1½ cups	crumbled feta cheese	375 mL
1 cup	diced red onion	250 mL
¾ cup	diced peeled celery (see Tips, left)	175 mL
2 tbsp	extra virgin olive oil	25 mL
1 tbsp	kosher salt	15 mL
1 tbsp	freshly ground black pepper	15 mL

1. *Vinaigrette:* In a bowl, whisk together lemon zest and juice, oil and garlic. Set aside.

2. *Salad:* On a baking sheet, roast tomatoes in preheated oven until soft and the skins begin to split, about 20 minutes. Transfer to a large bowl and add vinaigrette, chickpeas, feta, onion, celery, oil, salt and pepper. Toss gently to mix well. Cover and chill in the refrigerator for at least 2 hours or up to 1 week.

Nutrients per serving			
Calories	309	Dietary fiber	6.8 g
Protein	13.4 g	Sodium	564.3 mg
Total fat	15.6 g	Calcium	212.4 mg
Saturated fat	5.2 g	Iron	2.5 mg
Carbohydrates	29.0 g	Vitamin C	5.9 mg

Just for babies

As long as all the pieces are the appropriate size, this salad is a great choice for a toddler. It's loaded with nutrition and is a staple in the Wagman household. It makes a great snack served on toast or a whole romaine leaf. There you go — a meal to be eaten with your hands. What child wouldn't like that?

Nutrition Tip

Chickpeas, or garbanzo beans, are an important addition to a heart-healthy diet. They contain a significant amount of the vitamin folate, which helps break down the compound homocysteine. A buildup in homocysteine can damage blood vessel walls, leading to atherosclerosis and an increased risk of heart disease. Chickpeas are also very high in soluble fiber, which helps keep blood cholesterol under control, as well as insoluble fiber, which helps keep you regular.

Buy organic celery

Roasted Beet Salad

I love the sweetness of the beets and subtle tartness of the balsamic.

Makes about 4 cups (1 L)

- Preheat oven to 300°F (150°C)
- Baking sheet

3	beets (about 1 ½ lbs/750 g)	3
½ cup	balsamic vinegar	125 mL
¼ cup	extra virgin olive oil	50 mL
1 tsp	chopped fresh basil	5 mL
1 tsp	liquid honey	5 mL
Pinch	kosher salt	Pinch
Pinch	freshly ground black pepper	Pinch

Chef Jordan's Tips

When reducing small quantities of vinegar or sauces, I always begin with a hot pan; I find it saves a total of 2 to 3 minutes. That's time put to better use.

Don't serve this recipe to children under 1 year old, because it contains honey.

Nutrition Tip

Both the beet root and the beet greens have tremendous nutritional value. While the greens are rich in calcium and iron, the root contains a good amount of fiber and heart-healthy folic acid.

1. Place beets on a large piece of foil; tightly wrap and place on baking sheet. Roast in preheated oven until beets are fork tender, about 2½ hours. Let cool until cool enough to handle or, preferably, refrigerate overnight. Peel beets and coarsely chop.

2. Warm a saucepan over medium heat (see Tips, left). Add vinegar and bring to a boil. Boil until reduced by three-quarters, about 5 minutes. Let cool.

3. In a bowl, combine beets, vinegar, oil, basil, honey, salt and pepper. Serve immediately or transfer to an airtight container and refrigerate for up to 3 days.

Nutrients per serving (½ cup/125 mL)	
Calories 88	Dietary fiber . . . . . . 1.3 g
Protein . . . . 0.5 g	Sodium . . . . 59.4 mg
Total fat . . . . 6.0 g	Calcium . . . . 6.2 mg
Saturated fat. . . . . . 0.8 g	Iron . . . . 0.3 mg
Carbohydrates. . . . . 8.0 g	Vitamin C. . . . . . . 2.3 mg

Just for babies
Peel beets, dice and serve to toddlers.

Barley Salad with Apples and Sugar Snap Peas

A flavorful fresh salad filled with great textures everyone in the family will love.

Makes about 4 servings

■ ■ ■

Chef Jordan's Tips

This is your opportunity to clean your vegetable drawer. From broccoli and green beans to avocado, this salad will welcome any addition.

Nutrition Tip

Sugar snap peas are a cross between two types of peas, the green and the snow pea. They contain good amounts of immune-boosting vitamin C and bone-building vitamin K. When fresh peas are past their best, their sugars convert to starch. To make sure you are buying quality sugar-snap peas, snap one open to see if they are crisp, firm and bright green. Only store them for a few days unwashed in the refrigerator to enjoy maximum freshness.

Buy organic apples

1½ cups	cooked barley (see recipe, page 139)	375 mL
1 cup	finely diced cored apple	250 mL
½ cup	finely diced seeded peeled cucumber	125 mL
¼ cup	finely diced trimmed sugar snap peas	50 mL
1 tbsp	grated orange zest	15 mL
¼ cup	freshly squeezed orange juice	50 mL
¼ cup	extra virgin olive oil	50 mL
¼ cup	freshly grated Parmesan cheese	50 mL

1. In a bowl, combine barley, apple, cucumber, sugar snap peas, orange zest and juice, oil and Parmesan. Cover and refrigerate for at least 1 hour or up to 2 days.

Nutrients per serving

Calories	225	Dietary fiber	3.4 g
Protein	3.3 g	Sodium	67.6 mg
Total fat	13.4 g	Calcium	63.8 mg
Saturated fat	2.5 g	Iron	1.0 mg
Carbohydrates	23.7 g	Vitamin C	11.3 mg

Just for babies

Since all the ingredients in this salad are diced, it's a great dish to serve to a toddler.

Poached Whole Artichokes with Lemon Horseradish Aioli

This is a great way to enjoy whole artichokes. Bon appetit.

Makes about 2 servings

■ ■ ■

Chef Jordan's Tip

If you opened my refrigerator door you'd find a jar of store-bought mayonnaise, a good alternative to making your own. Don't get fooled into purchasing other emulsions sold in grocery chains that contain ingredients such as sugar and various seasonings. Real mayonnaise contains just oil, egg yolks, lemon juice or vinegar, and salt and pepper. In my opinion, the best are smooth and rich with little acidity, which allows me to add seasonings to suit the foodstuffs I'm serving. Homemade mayonnaise is a quite simple to make. Just combine 2 egg yolks, preferably free range (see Nutrition Tip, page 217) with 1 tsp (5 mL) Dijon mustard and whisk well.

10 cups	water	2.5 L
2	whole artichokes, (about 1½ lbs/750 g)	2
1	whole lemon, cut in half	1
2	bay leaves	2
1 tbsp	mustard seeds	15 mL
1 tbsp	white wine vinegar	15 mL
1 tsp	herbes de Provence	5 mL
1 tsp	kosher salt	5 mL
3	sprigs fresh thyme	3
	Lemon Horseradish Aioli (see recipe, page 206)	

1. Remove stems flush with lowest leaves so artichokes will stand upright. Peel outer portion of stems, leaving tender white core. Set stems aside.

2. Trim off top two-thirds of each artichoke and remove bright green leaves, exposing the whitish leaves. Plunge a spoon into the middle of choke, removing thorny middle leaves and exposing heart.

3. In a large pot over medium heat, bring water, artichokes, stems, lemon, bay leaves, mustard seeds, vinegar, herbes de Provence, salt and thyme to a boil. Reduce heat and simmer until stems are tender, about 10 minutes. Remove stems and transfer to a large bowl. Continue simmering artichokes until they are fork tender, about 30 minutes longer. Drain well, transfer to bowl containing stems, cover and refrigerate overnight. Serve with Lemon Horseradish Aioli for dipping.

Nutrients per serving

Calories	61	Dietary fiber	5.3 g
Protein	3.4 g	Sodium	1226.9 mg
Total fat	1.4 g	Calcium	76.5 mg
Saturated fat	0.0 g	Iron	2.6 mg
Carbohydrates	10.7 g	Vitamin C	14.5 mg

Just for babies

The stems make a great dish for older children. Serve them with carrot and celery sticks (both peeled, of course), and perhaps offer a mild dip, such as Cheddar Cheese Dip (see recipe, page 178).

Then slowly drizzle in ³⁄₄ cup (175 mL) extra virgin olive oil, whisking constantly until thick. Add a pinch of kosher salt and freshly ground black pepper.

Nutrition Tip

When using raw eggs, be aware that salmonella, a bacterium that can cause intestinal problems, can be a problem, particularly in eggs that come from large-scale farms. If you have any concerns about your egg supply, substitute ¹⁄₄ cup (50 mL) pasteurized liquid whole egg for the egg yolks called for in this recipe for homemade mayo. Pasteurized liquid whole egg product is available in cartons in the refrigerator section of most grocery stores. Do not use a liquid egg substitute product.

Honey Mustard-Glazed Salmon with Avocado

The combination of crisp salmon fillet and fresh avocado is a match made in heaven. I often serve this, or a variation, for lunch meetings with prospective customers for catering events, and guess what? The kids love this, too.

Makes 6 servings

■ ■ ■

Chef Jordan's Tips

Tossing sliced avocado in lemon juice prevents the avocado from turning brown, which can happen within a few moments. To preserve the beautiful green color of avocado, have the lemon juice in a bowl ready to toss before you peel and slice the avocado.

● **Preheat oven to 400°F (200°C)**

Honey Mustard Glaze

3 tbsp	Dijon mustard	45 mL
1 tbsp	liquid honey	15 mL
1 tsp	freshly ground black pepper	5 mL
1 tsp	chopped fresh chervil	5 mL
1 tsp	toasted sesame seeds	5 mL
½ tsp	mustard seeds	2 mL

Salmon

1 cup	avocado slices (see Tips, left)	250 mL
1 tbsp	freshly squeezed lemon juice	15 mL
1 tbsp	unsalted butter	15 mL
1 tbsp	extra virgin olive oil	15 mL
6	portions skin-on salmon fillets, (each about 4 oz/125 g)	6

1. *Honey Mustard Glaze:* In a bowl, whisk together mustard, honey, pepper, chervil, sesame seeds and mustard seeds. Set aside.

2. *Salmon:* In a bowl, combine avocado slices and lemon juice, tossing gently to evenly coat. Set aside.

3. In a skillet, heat butter and oil over high heat. Add salmon fillets, flesh side down, and cook until golden brown, about 4 minutes. Remove from heat. Flip fish and evenly coat seared side with the glaze. Roast in preheated oven, glazed side up, until firm to the touch and glaze is golden, about 5 minutes. Remove from heat and let rest for 2 to 4 minutes before serving.

4. On a platter, spread avocado slices out, creating a bed for the salmon. Place salmon on avocado and serve.

Nutrients per serving	
Calories 252	Dietary fiber . . . . . . 1.7 g
Protein . . . . 26.5 g	Sodium . . . . . . 276.2 mg
Total fat . . . . 12.6 g	Calcium . . . . 25.9 mg
Saturated fat. . . . . . 2.8 g	Iron . . . . 2.1 mg
Carbohydrates. . . . . 7.0 g	Vitamin C. . . . . . . 3.8 mg

Just for babies

Because this recipe contains honey, it should only be served to children who have passed their first birthday. Also, before serving any fish to a child, examine it closely for bones and remove any you find. That said, there's something magical about the combination of salmon and avocado, and if your children are old enough, they should be included in the festivities. Dice or mash their portion. Believe me, it will be an instant hit!

Nutrition Tip

Many people avoid avocados because of their high fat content. While they do contain a high percentage of fat, they are high in healthy fats such as oleic acid, which is also found in olive oil. This fat helps keep LDL (bad) cholesterol under control, among other benefits.

Grilled Portobello Mushroom Stack with Goat Cheese

One of my greatest challenges as a chef was cooking for vegetarians, even though I was a vegetarian for a number of years, myself. This dish, which is easy to make, kept my vegetarian customers happy and didn't require a lot of time or special ingredients. I'm sure you'll love this as much as my past customers did.

Makes about 4 servings

∎ ∎ ∎

Chef Jordan's Tips

If you come to our home you'll be guaranteed to find certain foodstuffs in the refrigerator — portobello mushrooms are certainly one of them. They are a versatile mushroom that can be used as both a side dish and the featured ingredient in any meal.

- Preheat barbecue to medium-high or 400°F (200°C)

4	portobello mushrooms, stems removed (about 1 lb/500 g)	4
1 tbsp	balsamic vinegar	15 mL
1 tbsp	extra virgin olive oil	15 mL
1 tsp	kosher salt, divided	5 mL
1 tsp	freshly ground black pepper, divided	5 mL
1 cup	Brussels Sprout Gratin (see recipe, page 85)	250 mL
½ cup	thinly sliced sweet onion, divided	125 mL
2	roasted red bell peppers, cut in half, divided	2
8	basil leaves	8
¼ cup	crumbled goat cheese, divided	50 mL
1 tsp	kosher salt, divided	5 mL
1 tsp	freshly ground black pepper, divided	5 mL

1. Holding mushroom stem side away from you, grab skin that hangs just beneath mushroom top and pull toward center to remove. Rotating mushroom in your hand, peel off strips until fully peeled. Repeat with remaining mushrooms. In a bowl, combine mushrooms, vinegar, olive oil and a pinch each of the salt and pepper.

2. Place mushrooms on a plate, peeled side down. Spread one-quarter of the Brussels Sprout Gratin on each mushroom. Top each with one-quarter of the onion, red peppers and basil and sprinkle with goat cheese. Season each layer with salt and pepper.

3. Place stacks on preheated barbecue and grill until mushrooms are soft and all ingredients are warmed through, about 10 minutes. Serve immediately or transfer to an airtight container and refrigerate for up to 3 days.

Nutrients per serving	
Calories 190	Dietary fiber ...... 4.4 g
Protein .... 9.1 g	Sodium ...... 657.5 mg
Total fat .... 10.3 g	Calcium ...... 134.0 mg
Saturated fat...... 4.4 g	Iron .... 1.2 mg
Carbohydrates.... 14.5 g	Vitamin C...... 78.4 mg

Just for babies

"Military style" is a term used in professional kitchens. It describes plating food, particularly for children, so that no ingredients touch one another. That's how I'd present this dish to my children. Separate all the ingredients, cut, dice, mash depending on their age, and allow them to pick and choose what to eat when. If you're serving this to a baby in the 9- to 12-month range, I'd suggest cutting off a piece and pulsing it in a food processor.

Nutrition Tip

Goat's milk cheese can often be tolerated by people who have an allergy or sensitivity to cheese made from cow's milk. Goat's milk cheese has approximately 10 per cent less lactose and its fat particles are about one-third the size of the fat particles in cow's milk, making it easier to break down and digest. It is also a good source of calcium, phosphorus and potassium.

Poppy Seed-Crusted Yellowfin Tuna with Roasted Shallots

I'm in love with this very simple and old-school recipe. The crispy texture of the seared poppy seeds contrasts beautifully with the smooth texture of the yellowfin (Ahi) tuna.

Makes 3 servings

Chef Jordan's Tips

There are only a few fish that substitute well for tuna in this dish, one of which is marlin. Served rare, it has a texture and flavor quite similar to tuna.

- Preheat oven to 350°F (180°C)
- Ovenproof skillet

¼ cup	poppy seeds	50 mL
1 tsp	kosher salt	5 mL
1 tsp	freshly ground pepper	5 mL
1 lb	yellowfin tuna loin, cut into 3 pieces (see Tips, left)	500 g
1 tbsp	extra virgin olive oil	15 mL
2	sprigs fresh thyme	2
1 cup	whole shallots, peeled	250 mL
1 tsp	minced garlic	5 mL
¼ cup	white wine	50 mL

1. In a bowl, combine poppy seeds, salt and pepper. Press into both sides of tuna. Set aside.

2. In ovenproof skillet, heat oil over medium-high heat. Add thyme and cook until there's no more "bubbling" around the thyme. Remove from pan and discard, leaving as much oil in the pan as possible. Add tuna and sear each side very quickly, about 30 seconds per side (the tuna should remain raw inside). Transfer tuna to a plate and keep warm.

3. Add shallots and garlic to the pan and sauté for a moment to evenly coat the shallots. Pour in wine. Transfer skillet to preheated oven. Roast shallots until soft, about 10 minutes.

4. To serve, thinly slice tuna loins and stack slices on a plate to resemble dominoes. Garnish with roasted shallots.

Nutrients per serving	
Calories 371	Dietary fiber . . . . . . 1.9 g
Protein . . . . 49.2 g	Sodium . . . . . . 828.5 mg
Total fat . . . . 11.9 g	Calcium. . . . . 208 mg
Saturated fat. . . . . . 1.7 g	Iron . . . . 3.4 mg
Carbohydrates. . . . 14.4 g	Vitamin C. . . . . . . 6.4 mg

Just for babies

I held off serving this dish to Jonah until he was about 13 months old because I was unsure about the texture of the poppy seeds and needed to tweak it a bit so the tuna would be cooked through. This is what I eventually came up with: In a small saucepan over medium heat, warm 1 tsp (5 mL) unsalted butter with about ¼ cup (50 mL) diced seared tuna and about 1 tbsp (15 mL), diced, of the roasted shallots. Heat until tuna is just cooked through, about 2 minutes. Remember, before serving any fish to a child, examine it closely for bones and remove any you find.

Nutrition Tip

There is considerable debate around fish, particularly tuna, and its potentially toxic contaminants versus its health benefits. In 2004 the Food and Drug Administration (FDA) and the Environmental Protection Agency (EPA) advised pregnant women and children to avoid large fish such as tuna, swordfish, shark, king mackerel and tilefish because they are likely to contain high levels of mercury. They recommended eating no more than 6 ounces (175 g) of these fish per week. However, these guidelines have recently been challenged by those who feel the nutritional benefits of eating fish outweigh any potential risks. Tuna is a nutrient-dense source of high-quality protein, selenium and vitamin B_{12}. It is also one of the best sources of omega-3 fats.

Israeli Couscous with Black Tiger Shrimp and Shrimp "Bisque"

If you're a shrimp lover, this recipe is for you!

Makes about
4 servings

■ ■ ■

Chef Jordan's Tips
In restaurants the goal is to maximize raw ingredients, creating as many dishes as you can with the "peripheral" cuts. After all, profit is not a dirty word. Whether it's beef tenderloin, which makes filet mignon and beef tartar (made from the "chain" meat") or carpaccio (made from the end cuts), chefs try to use everything. That's exactly how bisque was created; some chef had a surplus of shrimp shells and made a soup from them — a kickin' soup!

• Fine mesh strainer

Bisque

1 lb	black tiger shrimp	500 g
2 tbsp	extra virgin olive oil, divided	25 mL
1 cup	water	250 mL
1 cup	whole milk	250 mL
1 tsp	chipotle pepper powder	5 mL

Couscous

1 tbsp	minced fresh garlic	15 mL
½ cup	finely diced sweet onion	125 mL
¾ cup	chopped trimmed asparagus	175 mL
¾ cup	cherry tomatoes, halved	175 mL
2 cups	cooked Israeli couscous	500 mL
⅓ cup	freshly grated Parmesan cheese	75 mL

1. *Bisque:* Peel shrimp, reserving shells. Devein shrimp if necessary and coarsely chop. Set shrimp aside.

2. In a saucepan, heat 1 tbsp (15 mL) of the oil over medium heat. Add shrimp shells and sauté until they turn red, about 1 minute. Add water and bring to a boil. Reduce heat to low and simmer until most of the liquid has reduced, about 20 minutes. Add milk and chipotle powder and bring to a boil. Remove from heat. In a fine mesh strainer set over a bowl, strain out shrimp shells and discard. Set bisque aside.

224 NOT FOR ADULTS ONLY

3. *Couscous:* In another saucepan, heat remaining oil over medium-high heat. Add garlic and onion and sauté until onion is translucent, about 2 minutes. Add shrimp, asparagus and tomatoes and cook, stirring, until shrimp begin to turn red, about 2 minutes. Stir in bisque, couscous and Parmesan and bring to a boil. Serve immediately or transfer to an airtight container and refrigerate for up to 2 days.

Nutrients per serving			
Calories	436	Dietary fiber	2.3 g
Protein	49.0 g	Sodium	1437.3 mg
Total fat	13.2 g	Calcium	294.9 mg
Saturated fat	3.7 g	Iron	3.8 mg
Carbohydrates	26.3 g	Vitamin C	8.1 mg

Just for babies

Shellfish are among the more highly allergenic fish and should not be introduced to a child who may be allergy prone until he is about 3 years of age or even older. After that, this is a dish the entire family can enjoy together.

Nutrition Tip

Due to its appearance, couscous is often mistaken for a grain. In fact, it is part of the pasta family and is made from semolina wheat flour. Israeli couscous has larger spheres, the size of baby peas. Couscous is generally made from processed wheat flour, but you can search out couscous made from whole wheat, Kamut and spelt for the added vitamins, minerals and fiber that are present in whole grains.

Butter-Crusted Black Cod with Heirloom Tomatoes

I served this dish to my peers in Colorado Springs when we were celebrating our hotel's 4–diamond rating. It has a beautiful sweetness that makes it a decadent treat all year round.

Makes 6 servings

* * *

Chef Jordan's Tips

Treat the butter crust mixture like a compound butter. Wrap in plastic wrap and freeze for up to 6 months. To use, run a knife under hot water and wipe dry. Unwrap frozen mixture and cut to desired size. It makes a great topping for scallops, steak or tomatoes.

Get to know your local farmers or the people who staff your produce markets, because they can introduce you to the best seasonal foods, as well as varieties of fruits and vegetables that were grown years ago and are being resurrected because they taste far better than conventionally grown produce. One of the greatest relationships I forged was with a local farmer who grew heirloom vegetables.

- Preheat oven to 400°F (200°C)
- Ovenproof skillet

¹/₂ cup	fresh thyme sprigs, stems removed	125 mL
¹/₂ cup	diced whole wheat bread	125 mL
¹/₂ cup	unsalted butter	125 mL
¹/₄ cup	fresh parsley leaves	50 mL
¹/₄ cup	mascarpone cheese	50 mL
1 tsp	agave nectar	5 mL
Pinch	kosher salt	Pinch
Pinch	freshly ground black pepper	Pinch
2 lbs	skin-on black cod fillet, cut into 6 equal pieces	1 kg
2 cups	diced tomatoes, preferably heirloom	500 mL
¹/₂ cup	sweet white wine such as Sauternes or late-harvest Riesling	125 mL

1. In a food processor, combine thyme, bread, butter, parsley, mascarpone, agave nectar, salt and pepper and pulse until smooth. Transfer to a bowl (see Tips, left).

2. Using a butter knife, spread butter mixture over each piece of cod, flesh side only, fully encasing tops with crust. Place tomatoes in the bottom of ovenproof skillet and pour in wine. Place fish on top, buttered side up, pieces tightly together, so the fish resembles its original shape. Roast in preheated oven until crust is golden brown, about 25 minutes. Serve immediately or transfer to an airtight container and refrigerate for up to 2 days.

Nutrients per serving			
Calories	362	Dietary fiber	1.6 g
Protein	26.6 g	Sodium	298.9 mg
Total fat	24.5 g	Calcium	66.1 mg
Saturated fat	14.3 g	Iron	1.6 mg
Carbohydrates	8.6 g	Vitamin C	19.2 mg

Just for babies

What a great fish recipe to serve to children who have passed their first birthday — a fish that's high in good omega-3 fat content and beautiful tomatoes. What's not to love? Before serving any fish to a child, examine it closely for bones and remove any you find, then cut or dice this dish to suit their needs.

If you have the good fortune to come across heirloom tomatoes, buy them. These varieties, which are usually grown from saved seeds, rather than those that are industrially developed, are grown for one reason: flavor. Heirloom tomatoes range in color and size from very small "green zebras" to very large purple "brandywines." Although they are not the best looking tomatoes, the flavor is superb.

Nutrition Tip

Cod is an excellent low-calorie source of protein with good amounts of the heart- and brain-healthy omega-3 fatty acids. It also contains significant amounts of vitamins B_6 and B_{12}, both of which keep homocysteine levels in check. High homocysteine levels are associated with an increased risk of heart attack and stroke.

Salmon en Croute
with Arugula Salad

This is a great recipe — simple yet very elegant. Using puff pastry, which is an easy ingredient to work with, will make you look like a star.

**Makes about
4 servings**

■ ■ ■

Chef Jordan's Tips

There's no doubt, the best tools in the kitchen are your hands. For this salad, your hands are the only tool for the job. Arugula tends to bruise quite easily especially when tossed with tongs or spoons. A few swirls with your hands and each leaf will be coated with the dressing and blemish-free.

The peppery flavor of arugula is one you either love or, well, don't really care for. If you're looking for alternatives, thinly sliced romaine lettuce, dandelion leaves or sorrel are all great options as accompaniments to the salmon en croute.

- Preheat oven to 275°F (140°C)
- Baking sheet

¼ cup	extra virgin olive oil, divided	50 mL
1½ cups	sliced king oyster mushrooms	375 mL
2 tbsp	capers, rinsed and minced	25 mL
½	package (1 lb/500 g) frozen puff pastry, thawed	½
4	pieces skinless salmon fillet (each about 4 oz/125 g)	4
1 tbsp	grated lemon zest	15 mL
Pinch	kosher salt	Pinch
Pinch	freshly ground black pepper	Pinch
1	egg, beaten	1
2 cups	arugula	500 mL
2 tbsp	freshly squeezed lemon juice	25 mL

1. In a skillet, heat 2 tbsp (25 mL) of the oil over high heat. Add mushrooms and sauté until soft, about 3 minutes. Add capers and remove from heat. Let cool until warm to the touch and roughly chop. Set aside for later use.

2. If necessary, on lightly floured surface, roll out puff pastry into a 10-inch (25 cm) square. On a cutting board, cut pastry into four equal squares. Place one salmon fillet in the center of each square and sprinkle evenly with lemon zest. Divide mushroom mixture evenly on top of each and season with salt and pepper to taste.

3. Fold puff pastry over salmon and wrap edges under the package, keeping top smooth. Place on a baking sheet. Brush tops of pastry with egg. Bake in preheated oven until tops are golden brown, about 30 minutes.

4. In a bowl, combine remaining oil, arugula and lemon juice. Divide arugula mixture among four serving plates and place warm salmon en croute on top of salad.

Nutrients per serving	
Calories 837	Dietary fiber . . . . . . 3.0 g
Protein . . . . 46.5 g	Sodium . . . . . . 956.0 mg
Total fat . . . . 52.1 g	Calcium . . . . 49.0 mg
Saturated fat. . . . . 12.1 g	Iron . . . . 5.2 mg
Carbohydrates. . . . 45.1 g	Vitamin C. . . . . . . 7.0 mg

Just for babies

It's very important to make cooking and eating what you create fun. Whenever I made this recipe for Tamar and me, Jonah watched attentively and wanted to make his "present," too. (I assume because the salmon was wrapped.) It was only fair, after all. So we wrapped a small finger-size piece of salmon in the puff pastry and baked until it was golden brown, about 20 minutes. Remember, though, your child must have passed his first birthday to enjoy fish, and before serving any fish to a child, examine it closely for bones and remove any you find.

Nutrition Tip

Arugula has a split personality. As a "leafy green" it is rich in phytochemicals such as chlorophyll as well as vitamins, minerals and antioxidants. But it also acts as a cruciferous vegetable and as such contains anti-cancer compounds that stimulate detoxifying enzymes in the body.

Whole Roasted Chicken Stuffed with Lime and Green Onions

This is the greatest, simplest chicken recipe. Well, what are you waiting for?

Makes about 4 servings

■ ■ ■

Chef Jordan's Tips

The trick to evenly coating the flesh under the skin is to start with room temperature butter. Scoop half of the butter onto your fingers, push under the skin on one side of the breast and, using a waving motion similar to the windshield wipers on your car, wave back and forth until the side is fully coated. Repeat on the other breast.

I really love the flavor cooked green onions impart to the chicken, but in their absence, I'll choose the whites of leeks or whole bulbs of garlic cut in half to expose the flesh.

- Preheat oven to 450°F (230°C)
- Large ovenproof skillet or roasting pan

1	whole chicken (about 3 lbs/1.5 kg)	1
1 tbsp	unsalted butter, at room temperature	15 mL
1	lime, cut in half	1
6	green onions, trimmed, divided	6
1 tsp	kosher salt, divided	5 mL
1 tsp	freshly ground black pepper, divided	5 mL

1. Place chicken on a plate breast side up. Separate the skin from the breast meat by sliding your fingers underneath the skin and moving them from side-to-side without removing the skin. This will create a "pocket". Using your fingers, spread butter under skin covering as much of the breast as possible.

2. Open cavity of chicken and stuff with lime, half of the green onions and a pinch each of the salt and pepper. Tie legs together to close cavity and tuck wings underneath. Season outside of bird with remaining salt and pepper. Place remaining green onions in the bottom of a large ovenproof skillet and place chicken on top, breast side up (this prevents the chicken from sticking to the pan).

3. Roast in preheated oven for 35 minutes. Reduce heat to 350°F (180°C) and roast until juices run clear when thigh is pierced and a thermometer inserted in the thigh registers 165°F (75°C), about 40 minutes. Transfer to a cutting board, tent with foil and let rest for 15 minutes before serving.

Calories	531	Dietary fiber	0.6 g
Protein	43.0 g	Sodium	648.7 mg
Total fat	37.6 g	Calcium	33.7 mg
Saturated fat	11.7 g	Iron	2.9 mg
Carbohydrates	3.0 g	Vitamin C	19.4 mg

Just for babies

This recipe, which contains 3 ingredients, is ideal for babies as young as 9 months to enjoy so long as they have been introduced to onions and chicken separately. Although citrus is usually reserved until your baby has passed the 12-month mark due to potential allergies, the amount here is so small, it's not likely to be a problem.

Nutrition Tip

You can rest assured you are investing in your health if you buy free-range poultry. Free-range farming is an old-school method of husbandry that allows animals to roam freely. Commercially produced chickens can suffer from many conditions found in "high-density housing." Look for 100% certified organic, free-range chickens that will also have been exposed to fresh air, sunlight, and insects (although this may sound odd, insects are a good protein source and a normal part of a free-range chicken's diet) and be hormone-, pesticide- and antibiotic-free.

Citrus BBQ-Glazed Baby Back Ribs

My first and only attempt at owning a restaurant was a success due to this sauce, which can also be used as a marinade. It became an overnight hit with my customers, as it will in your home. Enjoy.

Makes about 2 servings

■ ■ ■

Chef Jordan's Tips

Most families have their favorite barbecue sauce, whether it is store bought or a recipe handed down through generations. By all means use the version you love most.

On the weekends in the summertime, I cook baby back ribs on indirect heat on the barbecue for about 5 hours. To cook on indirect heat, you need a gas barbecue with at least 2 burners or, use a charcoal grill. Preheat your barbecue to 200°F (100°C) on one side (or push the coals to one side) and place the ribs on the unlit side. Cooking slowly imparts a remarkable flavor that can't be artificially created.

- Preheat oven to 300°F (150°C)
- Large ovenproof skillet or roasting pan

¾ cup	barbecue sauce (see Tips, left)	175 mL
½ cup	minced green onions	125 mL
¼ cup	freshly squeezed lemon juice	50 mL
¼ cup	freshly squeezed orange juice	50 mL
1 tbsp	liquid honey	15 mL
1	rack pork baby back ribs, cut in half (about 1½ lbs/750 g)	1

1. In a bowl, combine barbecue sauce, green onions, lemon juice, orange juice and honey.
2. In large ovenproof skillet, combine ribs and sauce, rubbing sauce into ribs with your hands, getting every nook and cranny covered.
3. Bake in preheated oven until ribs are caramelized and meat is beginning to separate from bone, about 85 minutes.

Just for babies

If your baby has passed his first birthday, he will love these ribs, minus the bones, of course. Remove the meat from the bone and chop or dice the meat for Baby. For older children, create a boneless rib for them to eat with their hands as you do. With a knife remove the meat from both sides of the rib in one strip and cut away any potentially dangerous pockets of fat. (I'm referring to the potential choking hazard.)

Nutrition Tip

Be aware that there are nutritional considerations when selecting cuts of meat. Leaner cuts of meat, such as the foreshank or a whole leg, have a higher moisture and protein content, while the cuts with higher fat content, such as the ribs, shoulder and loin, have less of both. It's the fat content in baby back ribs that gives them such a succulent taste and makes them so high in calories. The prepared barbecue sauce is responsible for the high sodium content. Make sure you add lots of green vegetables and whole grains when you enjoy this and other meat recipes. You'll want to round out the meal by expanding the range of nutrients it provides and ensure that you get an adequate amount of fiber.

Oven-Roasted Cornish Hen with Sage

Not your average chicken. Cornish hen has a delicate flavor that is very appealing.

Makes about 2 servings

■ ■ ■

Nutrition Tip

In fresh or dry forms or in teas, sage is used as an astringent to treat excessive perspiration, night sweats and diarrhea. It is very well known as an aid for drying up unwanted breast milk when mothers want to stop nursing. Sage is also antibacterial and antiviral and makes a wonderful gargle for sore throats.

- Preheat oven to 450°F (230°C)
- Ovenproof skillet

1	Cornish hen (about 1½ lbs/750 g)	1
1 tbsp	freshly ground spice mixture (see page 243)	15 mL
6	sage leaves	6
1 tsp	unsalted butter	5 mL
½ tsp	extra virgin olive oil	2 mL

1. Season hen with spice mixture, rubbing the spices into the skin and using your hands to thoroughly coat the whole bird. Stuff sage into cavity. Tie legs to close cavity and tuck wings under back.

2. In ovenproof skillet, heat butter and oil over high heat. Add hen, breast side down, and sear until nicely browned, about 3 minutes. Turn hen over and transfer skillet to preheated oven. Roast until juices run clear when thigh is pierced, about 30 minutes. Transfer to a cutting board and let rest for 7 to 10 minutes before cutting.

Nutrients per serving	
Calories 461	Dietary fiber . . . . . . 0.0 g
Protein . . . . 75.2 g	Sodium . . . . . . 255.3 mg
Total fat . . . . 15.4 g	Calcium . . . . 45.6 mg
Saturated fat. . . . . . 4.5 g	Iron . . . . 2.8 mg
Carbohydrates. . . . . 0.0 g	Vitamin C. . . . . . . 2.3 mg

Just for babies

If your baby has been introduced to poultry, purée some for him to enjoy.

Aging Meat

How beef is aged plays a very important role in its flavor and tenderness. There are two ways to age beef: dry and wet. Wet aging is done in a vacuum-sealed bag, which doesn't allow the meat to lose moisture. However, it develops an average flavor profile. Dry aging is done in a temperature- and moisture-controlled setting for a minimum of two weeks. Most dry-aged beef is so tender it can be cut with a spoon, and the depth of flavor is far superior to wet-aged meats. Since dry aging is time consuming and significant moisture is drawn from the cut of beef, which means it weighs less than wet-aged meat, this process is quite costly. Consequently, it is not the preferred method of most supermarkets and many butchers. But it is certainly the method most higher-end restaurants prefer, which is why your steak is likely to taste better when you eat out than it does at home.

The next time you visit your butcher, ask them about the method they use. If they dry age their meat, wonderful. But if they use the wet method, try a little taste test. Find out where you can buy a dry-aged steak and cook it alongside one of theirs that is wet aged. I think you'll find a big difference between the two and will become a convert to dry-aged beef.

"Cassoulet" of Black Eyed Peas, Chorizo Sausage and NY Steak

Some of my mentors would be offended, but this twist on a classic French dish is one of my family's favorites on a cool fall or winter's evening.

Makes 4 servings

∎ ∎ ∎

Chef Jordan's Tips

Feel free to use your bean of choice, from white or red kidney to larger fava beans, instead of the black-eyed peas. All work well. Be sure to alter your cooking times to suit the bean you're using.

For best results, I recommend cooking the steak to medium-rare. It will continue to cook after removal from the liquid and will also cook under the broiler.

● Individual casserole dishes (each about 1½ cups/375 mL)

1 cup	soaked dried black-eyed peas (see page 77), drained and rinsed	250 mL
6 cups	water	1.5 L
2	cloves garlic, minced	2
2	fresh chorizo sausages (about 10 oz/300 g)	2
1	New York strip loin steak (about 1 lb/500 g)	1
1 cup	finely diced peeled parsnips	250 mL
½ cup	diced peeled turnip	125 mL
1	bay leaf	1
1 tsp	kosher salt	5 mL
Pinch	chipotle pepper powder	Pinch
2 tbsp	coarsely chopped chives	25 mL
1 tbsp	red wine vinegar	15 mL
1 cup	freshly grated Parmesan cheese, divided	250 mL

1. In a large saucepan, combine peas, water and garlic. Bring to a boil over medium heat. Reduce heat to low and simmer until the peas are tender, about 30 minutes.

2. Add sausages, steak, parsnips, turnip, bay leaf, salt and chipotle powder and simmer until sausage is fully cooked, about 10 minutes (the steak will be a perfect medium-rare). Using tongs, transfer the sausage and steak to a cutting board, leaving beans and vegetables in the pan. Let meat rest for a minimum of 4 minutes. Thinly slice the steak across the grain and cut sausage into slices.

3. Meanwhile, continue to cook the beans until they reach a creamy consistency, 10 to 15 minutes. Remove from heat and stir in chives and vinegar.

4. Preheat broiler. Spoon bean mixture into dishes and drape sliced steak and sausage over top of the beans. Sprinkle Parmesan cheese evenly over top of each dish. Broil until cheese is golden brown, 3 to 5 minutes.

Nutrients per serving	
Calories 744	Dietary fiber . . . . . . 4.9 g
Protein . . . . 68.4 g	Sodium . . . . . . 843.2 mg
Total fat . . . . 42.4 g	Calcium . . . . . . 309.5 mg
Saturated fat. . . . . 17.3 g	Iron . . . . 5.3 mg
Carbohydrates. . . . 19.0 g	Vitamin C. . . . . . 10.6 mg

Just for babies
Cooled and diced, this zesty mélange is suitable for children who have passed their first birthday. Make sure they have been introduced to all the ingredients individually before they sample the dish.

Nutrition Tip
A typical adult in North America consumes an average of 10 to 15 grams of fiber per day. The recommended fiber dosage for good health is more than double that. Legumes — dried beans, peas and lentils — are an excellent source of soluble fiber, which moves slowly as a gel through the digestive system. With regular consumption, this type of fiber can help reduce cholesterol levels and maintain healthy blood sugar levels.

Veal Rib Chops with Fresh Corn and Asparagus Succotash

WARNING! Ladies and gentleman lock your doors and windows or your neighbors will be kicking them down once the smell of this dish permeates the streets. Good luck. You've been warned.

Makes about 2 servings

■ ■ ■

Chef Jordan's Tips

To season or not to season? I've heard for years, from every chef I've trained with, season everything — words I choose to live by. One exception these days is salt. I find that when I season with salt I create a layer between the heat source and the meat, making it very difficult to achieve that caramelization I speak about over and over again. Salt will leach the natural juices out of meat — by salting it in advance of searing you will create a layer of water on top of the meat, water that will first have to evaporate before allowing the meat to sear. These days I salt the meat as soon as it finishes cooking.

● Preheat oven to 400°F (200°C)
● Ovenproof skillet

2	bone-in veal rib chops (about 1¼ lbs/625 g)	2
½ tsp	freshly ground black pepper	2 mL
1 tsp	unsalted butter	5 mL
1 tsp	extra virgin olive oil	5 mL
2	sprigs fresh thyme	2
1¾ cups	corn kernels	425 mL
½ cup	coarsely chopped trimmed asparagus	125 mL
2	cloves garlic, minced	2
½ tsp	kosher salt	2 mL

1. On a plate, season veal chops on both sides with pepper.

2. In ovenproof skillet, heat butter and oil over high heat. Add veal chops and sear until golden brown, about 5 minutes. Flip chops and add thyme. Transfer skillet to preheated oven and roast for about 10 minutes for medium-rare, 15 minutes for medium or 25 minutes for well-done. Remove from heat and transfer chops to a plate, leaving sprigs of thyme in the pan. Set the veal chops aside to rest. Season with salt.

3. In the hot skillet, combine corn, asparagus, garlic and salt. Return skillet to oven. Roast until corn is tender, about 8 minutes.

4. Spoon the corn mixture in a pile in the center of a platter and place chops on top.

Nutrients per serving

Calories	884	Dietary fiber	4.7 g
Protein	80.2 g	Sodium	713.1 mg
Total fat	49.6 g	Calcium	55.6 mg
Saturated fat	18.7 g	Iron	4.7 mg
Carbohydrates	28.9 g	Vitamin C	13.5 mg

Just for babies

If your baby has been introduced to the individual ingredients separately, by all means cut off a piece of the chop and purée for babies as young as those in the 6- to 9-month range. If diced appropriately it will make a delicious meal for a toddler.

Nutrition Tip

Asparagus contains a good amount of fiber and is relatively high in protein for a vegetable. It also contains sulfur, which helps the liver with its detoxification jobs, and folic acid to help with heart health. Some people notice that their urine has an unusual smell after they eat this springtime vegetable. It comes from the amino acid asparagine, which is named after this vegetable.

Sliced NY Steak with Mushroom Duxelles and Fresh Horseradish

This meal is easy and so good that you and your family will think you've hired a 5-star chef to cook the meal! Enjoy it as a splurge.

Makes 2 servings

■ ■ ■

Chef Jordan's Tips

One of the most important lessons I've learned throughout my years of cooking is to rest meat and poultry after cooking. The rule of thumb is the amount of resting time should equal one-third the cooking time. For example, if a steak takes you 30 minutes to cook, rest the meat for a minimum of 10 minutes prior to slicing. This gives juices ample time to disperse throughout the meat instead of ending up in a puddle on your plate.

1 tbsp	unsalted butter, divided	15 mL
1½ cups	minced mushrooms	375 mL
2	cloves garlic, minced	2
1	bay leaf	1
1 tbsp	Dijon mustard	15 mL
1 tsp	extra virgin olive oil	5 mL
1	New York strip loin steak (about 1 lb/500 g)	1
¼ cup	chicken stock or water	50 mL
1 tbsp	crumbled blue cheese	15 mL
1 tbsp	freshly grated horseradish or prepared horseradish, drained	15 mL

1. In a saucepan, melt 1 tsp (5 mL) of the butter over medium heat. Add mushrooms, garlic and bay leaf and sauté until water in mushrooms has evaporated and mushrooms are "dry," about 10 minutes. Stir in mustard, discard bay leaf and set aside.

2. In a skillet, heat remaining butter and the oil over medium-high heat. Add steak and sear until nicely browned, about 10 minutes. Flip steak and continue to cook another 5 minutes for medium-rare, 10 minutes for medium or 15 minutes for well done. Transfer to a cutting board and let rest.

3. Return the skillet to medium-low heat. Add chicken stock and bring to a boil. With a wooden spoon or spatula, scrape the bottom of the pan, releasing brown bits stuck to the bottom. Stir in blue cheese. Boil until sauce has reduced by half, about 5 minutes.

4. Thinly slice steak across the grain, lay it out on warmed serving plates and sprinkle with horseradish. Spoon sauce onto the plate directly beside the steak. Serve mushroom duxelles in a small dish on the side.

Nutrients per serving	
Calories 576	Dietary fiber . . . . . . 2.0 g
Protein . . . . 80.8 g	Sodium . . . . . . 429.0 mg
Total fat . . . . 24.3 g	Calcium . . . . . . 87.8 mg
Saturated fat. . . . . 10.3 g	Iron . . . . 5.3 mg
Carbohydrates. . . . . 5.2 g	Vitamin C. . . . . . . 5.5 mg

Just for babies

Before plating this dish for Mom and Dad, set aside a portion for Baby — this is suitable even for those in the 6- to 9-month age group if they have been introduced to all the ingredients individually. Purée. For older children, cut the meat into an appropriately sized dice.

Nutrition Tip

Horseradish is a member of the cabbage family. This pungent root is known as a cholagogue, a compound that stimulates the gallbladder to release its storage of bile. It is important for the gallbladder to receive these strong stimulant signals so that the bile does not become sluggish and congested, leading to an increased risk of gallstones.

Spice-Rubbed Rack of Lamb

Once you've made this recipe, it will become part of your weekly repertoire. It reminds me of lamb lollipops!

Makes about 2 servings

▪ ▪ ▪

Nutrition Tip
Coriander and cumin seeds have a long tradition as healing spices. Both contain volatile essential oils that act as digestive aids and make them effective carminatives. This means that the oils affect the digestive system by relaxing the stomach muscles, reducing the production of gas and moving material through the intestines in a timely manner. Whenever possible, buy whole seeds because they retain these helpful oils longer than those that are ground.

- Preheat oven to 450°F (230°C)
- Ovenproof skillet

1	rack of lamb (about 8 oz/250 g)	1
1 tsp	freshly ground spice mixture (see page 243)	5 mL
1 tbsp	extra virgin olive oil	15 mL
Pinch	kosher salt	Pinch

1. Place lamb on a plate. Grind spice mixture over top of lamb, evenly distributing spices; set aside.

2. In ovenproof skillet, heat oil over medium-high heat. Add lamb, skin-side down, and sear until a nice crust has developed, about 5 minutes. Transfer skillet to the oven and roast until lamb is firm to the touch, about 15 minutes for medium-rare. Remove from heat; rest a minimum of 10 minutes before slicing (see Tips, page 240). Slice into chops, season with salt and serve. Enjoy immediately.

Nutrients per serving			
Calories	392	Dietary fiber	0.0 g
Protein	18.7 g	Sodium	477.1 mg
Total fat	34.5 g	Calcium	14.7 mg
Saturated fat	14.5 g	Iron	1.52 mg
Carbohydrates	0.0 g	Vitamin C	0.0 mg

Just for babies
If your baby has been introduced to lamb and these spices, a puréed version of this recipe could be served to babies in the 6- to 9-month age range. If you're concerned about the spices, cut from the unseasoned part of the meat.

Make Your Own Spice Blend

In the professional kitchens I've worked in, and as a home cook, I enjoy the flavors created by combining different spices, which I grind into a blend and use to season food. I have so many spice mixtures labeled and ready to go for everyday use in our kitchen that I think Tamar is getting tired of all the peppermills cluttering the counter. The spice mixture I use to make this rack of lamb is equal parts whole, untoasted coriander seeds, cumin seeds and fennel seeds. I keep it in a grinder and grind it just as I need it, which provides the freshest flavor. If you don't have a spice grinder, put the spices in a mortar and grind with a pestle, or combine them on a cutting board, lay a clean kitchen cloth on top and use a rolling pin, the bottom of a wine bottle or the back of a sauté pan to grind them.

I have two general rules that can be applied to using spices: Don't toast the spices if you're using them on raw food that is going to be cooked (if I'm making a tartar, which is raw, I'd want the spices to be toasted), but toast them to bring out the flavor when seasoning food that is already cooked. For example, if I'm creating a mixture to season a steak before it's cooked, I won't toast the spices before adding them to the peppermill. But if I wanted a spice blend to use on top of smoked salmon for a family brunch, I'd toast the spices first. To toast whole spices, heat in a dry skillet over medium heat, stirring constantly, just until they release their fragrance. Let them cool before adding to the grinder. Toasting brings their natural oils to the surface, dramatically enhancing their flavor.

It's easy to make your own blends built around your favorite spices. Start by thinking about what to pair with black peppercorns, for example, add some cumin seeds or coriander seeds to the peppercorns.

My favorite spice mixture is the following: 1 tbsp (15 mL) each cumin seeds, coriander seeds, hot pepper flakes and mustard seeds.

Library and Archives Canada Cataloguing in Publication

Wagman, Jordan
    Easy gourmet baby food : 150 recipes for homemade goodness /
Jordan Wagman & Jill Hillhouse.

Includes index.
ISBN 978-0-7788-0182-5

1. Cookery (Baby foods). 2. Infants—Nutrition. I. Hillhouse, Jill II. Title.

TX740.W33 2008   641.5'6222   C2007-907054-X

Index

a

Acorn Squash Purée, 43
ADHD, 23
agave nectar/syrup, 191
  Cheesecake Soufflé, 190
  Cranberry Phyllo "Pinwheels", 196
  Frozen Blueberry Sorbet, 183
  Mini Sweet Potato Muffins with Maple Syrup
    Glaze, 176
  Short-Grain Brown Rice Pudding with
    Chocolate Wafers, 193
Alaskan Halibut en Papillote, 152
allergies, 22, 24–25
allicin, 88
allium (onion) family, 83
amino acids, 74, 104, 165
apples, 35, 116, 162, 186
  Apple and Fig Brown Rice Cereal, 56
  Apple and Strawberry Compote, 118
  Apple Medley, 35
  Applesauce, My Mom's, 186
  Barley Salad with Apples and Sugar Snap
    Peas, 215
  Berry-Glazed Fig Tart, 194
  Chicken with Caramelized Apples, 162
  Fennel and Apple–Stuffed Pork Chops, 158
  Red Cabbage, Fennel and Apple Purée, 96
  Red Lentil and Apple, 71
  Roasted Apple, Blueberry and Pear, 58
  Roasted Beet Salad, 214
  Roasted Summer Fruit (tip), 120
  Sautéed Chard with Apples, 102
  Strawberries with Granny Smith Apples, 116
  Whole-Grain Oat Cereal with Grapes
    (variation), 53
apricots, 37
  Apricot Acorn Squash Purée, 60
  Fresh Apricot Purée, 37
  Oven-Roasted Chicken with Dried Apricots,
    106
  Whole-Grain Oat Cereal with Grapes
    (variation), 53

artichokes, 125
  Oven-Roasted Artichokes, 124
  Poached Whole Artichokes with Lemon
    Horseradish Aioli, 216
arugula, 229
  Salmon en Croute with Arugula Salad (tip),
    228
  White Navy Bean and Beef Tenderloin Purée
    (variation), 76
asparagus, 129, 239
  Alaskan Halibut en Papillote, 152
  Asparagus and Roasted Tomato, 128
  Grilled Asparagus with Three Cheeses, 134
  Israeli Couscous with Black Tiger Shrimp
    and Shrimp "Bisque", 224
  Veal Rib Chops with Fresh Corn and
    Asparagus Succotash, 238
avocado, 182, 218
  Avocado, Carrot and Cucumber Purée, 70
  Grilled Chicken and Avocado, 75
  Guacamole, 182
  Honey Mustard–Glazed Salmon with
    Avocado, 218

b

baby food. *See also* food
  for 6 to 9 months, 32–76
  for 9 to 12 months, 80–111
  equipment for, 28
  preparing, 26–27, 71
  processed, 14–15
  storing and freezing, 27–28
  for toddlers, 114–67
bacon, 93
  Brussels Sprouts with Bacon, 93
  Corn and Chickpea Chowder, 127
  Oven-Roasted Artichokes, 124
bananas, 34
  Applesauce, My Mom's (tip), 186
  Banana and Blueberry Purée, 67
  Millet Cereal with Crushed Bananas and
    Sour Cream, 90

bananas (*continued*)
Mini Chocolate Chunk Banana Sandwiches, 180
Quinoa and Banana Purée, 54
Roasted Banana Purée, 34
Tofu, Bosc Pears and Banana, 57
Whole-Grain Oat Crêpes with Warm Bananas, 146
Barbecued Corn, Best-Ever, 136
barley and barley flour, 51, 52, 139
Barley Salad with Apples and Sugar Snap Peas, 215
Basic Pearled Barley, 139
Classic Beef and Barley Stew, 156
Simple Barley Cereal, 52
Warm Barley with Fresh Herbs and Parmesan Cheese, 140
Basic Pearled Barley, 139
Basic Quinoa, 48
Basic Sweet-and-Sour Sauce, 209
basil, 61
Asparagus and Roasted Tomato, 128
Citrus Fruit Salad with Fresh Basil, 122
Creamy Brown Rice and Fresh Basil, 142
Eggplant Parmesan, The Best, 84
Green Bean Purée with Fresh Basil, 61
Grilled Portobello Mushroom Stack with Goat Cheese, 220
Mediterranean Fried Eggplant, 86
Oven-Roasted Cherry Tomato Purée, 94
Oven-Roasted Red Peppers, 208
Ratatouille Vegetables, 101
Turkey Meatloaf, Gramma Jean's, 164
Warm Pineapple with Cottage Cheese and Basil, 119
Zucchini and Basil Purée, 64
beans, 77, 105
"Cassoulet" of Black-Eyed Peas, Chorizo Sausage and NY Steak (tip), 236
Fresh Soy Bean Hummus, 103
White Bean and Fennel Purée, 104
White Navy Bean and Beef Tenderloin Purée, 76
beef, 235
Beef Tenderloin and Dates, 110
"Cassoulet" of Black-Eyed Peas, Chorizo Sausage and NY Steak, 236
Classic Beef and Barley Stew, 156

Sliced NY Steak with Mushroom Duxelles and Fresh Horseradish, 240
White Navy Bean and Beef Tenderloin Purée, 76
beets, 46, 214
Roasted Beet Purée, 46
Roasted Beet Salad, 214
bell peppers, 91, 205, 208
Alaskan Halibut en Papillote, 152
Corn and Chickpea Chowder, 127
Egg and Sweet Pepper Fried Rice, 91
Grilled Portobello Mushroom Stack with Goat Cheese, 220
Oven-Roasted Red Peppers, 208
Pacific Salmon Cakes, 155
Ratatouille Vegetables, 101
Roasted Red Pepper Vinaigrette, 205
Turkey Meatloaf, Gramma Jean's, 164
berries. *See also specific types of berries*
Berry-Glazed Fig Tart, 194
Strawberries with Granny Smith Apples (tip), 116
The Best Eggplant Parmesan, 84
Best-Ever Barbecued Corn, 136
beta-carotene, 39, 42, 68
blood sugar, 177
blueberries, 38, 63, 183
Banana and Blueberry Purée, 67
Berry-Glazed Fig Tart, 194
Blueberry Purée, 38
Frozen Blueberry Sorbet, 183
Honeydew, Blueberry and Mint Purée, 62
Plum and Blueberry Purée, 63
Roasted Apple, Blueberry and Pear, 58
Roasted Summer Fruit, 120
Watermelon, Peach and Blueberry Purée, 69
Bok Choy with Fresh Ginger, 92
Bosc Pear Purée, 36
bottle feeding, 32
brassica (cabbage) family, 85, 96, 137
bread (as ingredient)
Brussels Sprout Gratin (variation), 85
Butter-Crusted Black Cod with Heirloom Tomatoes, 226
French Toast with Fresh Peaches and Peachy Maple Syrup, 148
breastfeeding, 32, 129

broccoli
  Broccoli, Potato and Spinach Pie, 133
  Broccoli Purée, 40
  Soft Polenta with Cheddar Cheese and
    Broccoli Florets, 143
bromelain, 119
Brown Rice Cereal, 50
Brussels sprouts
  Brussels Sprout Gratin, 85
  Brussels Sprouts with Bacon, 93
  Grilled Portobello Mushroom Stack with
    Goat Cheese, 220
butter, 136
  Barbecued Corn, Best-Ever, 136
  Butter-Crusted Black Cod with Heirloom
    Tomatoes, 226

C

cabbage
  Pork with Red Cabbage, 160
  Red Cabbage, Fennel and Apple Purée, 96
  Red Cabbage with Duck Confit, 167
calcium, 40, 178
cane sugar, 185
capers
  Caper and Lemon Remoulade, 207
  Lemon Horseradish Aioli, 206
  Salmon en Croute with Arugula Salad, 228
Caramelized Parsnip Purée, 47
carbohydrates, complex, 45
carotenoids, 68, 182, 204. See also
    beta-carotene; lycopene
carrots
  Avocado, Carrot and Cucumber Purée, 70
  Basic Sweet-and-Sour Sauce, 209
  Carrot and Split Pea Purée, 68
  Carrot Purée, 44
  Israeli Couscous with Grated Carrots and
    Chives, 144
  Nectarine and Carrot Purée, 59
  Quick Mushroom Soup, 126
  Red Potato Salad with Cheddar Cheese and
    Boiled Eggs, 135
  Roasted Chicken Stock, 202
  Vegetable Stock, 201
  White Navy Bean and Beef Tenderloin Purée,
    76

"Cassoulet" of Black-Eyed Peas, Chorizo
    Sausage and NY Steak, 236
cauliflower
  Cauliflower and Chickpea Chowder, 66
  Cauliflower and Parsnip Purée, 65
  Millet and Cauliflower with Fresh Oregano,
    141
  Oven-Roasted Cauliflower with Fresh Herbs,
    137
  Salmon, Potato and Cauliflower, 154
celery
  Chickpea, Grape Tomato and Feta Salad,
    212
  Cucumber Salad with Smoked Salmon, 210
  Roasted Chicken Stock, 202
  Vegetable Stock, 201
Celery Root and Chicken Purée, 72
cereals, 48–56, 89, 90
cheese. See also specific types of cheese (below)
  Blueberry Purée (variation), 38
  Butter-Crusted Black Cod with Heirloom
    Tomatoes, 226
  Cheesecake Soufflé, 190
  Chicken and Red Lentils (variation), 74
  Chickpea, Grape Tomato and Feta Salad,
    212
  Grilled Asparagus with Three Cheeses, 134
  Sliced NY Steak with Mushroom Duxelles
    and Fresh Horseradish, 240
  Turkey Meatloaf, Gramma Jean's, 164
  Warm Pineapple with Cottage Cheese and
    Basil, 119
cheese, Cheddar, 143
  Asparagus and Roasted Tomato (variation),
    128
  Cheddar Cheese Dip, 178
  Grilled Chicken and Avocado (variation), 75
  Red Potato Salad with Cheddar Cheese and
    Boiled Eggs, 135
  Soft Polenta with Cheddar Cheese and
    Broccoli Florets, 143
cheese, goat, 221
  Broccoli, Potato and Spinach Pie (variation),
    133
  Grilled Portobello Mushroom Stack with
    Goat Cheese, 220
  Millet Cereal with Crushed Bananas and
    Sour Cream (tip), 90

cheese, goat (*continued*)
  Oven-Roasted Cauliflower with Fresh Herbs, 137
  Plum and Blueberry Purée (variation), 63
cheese, Parmesan, 140
  Barley Salad with Apples and Sugar Snap Peas, 215
  Basic Quinoa (variation), 48
  Broccoli, Potato and Spinach Pie, 133
  Broccoli Purée (variation), 40
  Brussels Sprout Gratin, 85
  "Cassoulet" of Black-Eyed Peas, Chorizo Sausage and NY Steak, 236
  "Chips and Salsa" — Parmesan Cheese Crisps with Plum Salsa, 174
  Chive Parsley "Pistou" (tip), 99
  Diced Potato Gratin, 87
  Eggplant Parmesan, The Best, 84
  "Fish Sticks", World's Best, 150
  Israeli Couscous with Black Tiger Shrimp and Shrimp "Bisque", 224
  "Mac and Cheese", Jonah's, 138
  Mediterranean Fried Eggplant, 86
  Oven-Roasted Artichokes, 124
  Warm Barley with Fresh Herbs and Parmesan Cheese, 140
  Zucchini and Basil Purée (variation), 64
Cheesecake Soufflé, 190
cherries
  Pork with Red Cabbage, 160
  Summer Cherry and Quinoa, 89
chicken. *See also* poultry
  Celery Root and Chicken Purée, 72
  Chicken and Red Lentils, 74
  Chicken with Caramelized Apples, 162
  Chicken with Roasted Butternut Squash and Leeks, 108
  Grilled Chicken and Avocado, 75
  Onion Soup with Cornish Hen (tip), 163
  Oven-Roasted Chicken with Dried Apricots, 106
  Potato, Parsnip and Chicken Soup with Chive Parsley "Pistou", 98
  Roasted Chicken Stock, 202
  Whole Roasted Chicken Stuffed with Lime and Green Onions, 230
chickpeas, 66, 77, 213
  Cauliflower and Chickpea Chowder, 66

Chickpea, Grape Tomato and Feta Salad, 212
  Corn and Chickpea Chowder, 127
  Fresh Soy Bean Hummus, 103
"Chips and Salsa" — Parmesan Cheese Crisps with Plum Salsa, 174
chives
  "Cassoulet" of Black-Eyed Peas, Chorizo Sausage and NY Steak, 236
  Chive Parsley "Pistou", 99
  Cucumber Salad with Smoked Salmon, 210
  Israeli Couscous with Grated Carrots and Chives, 144
  Turnip and Parsnip "Smash" (variation), 95
chlorophyll, 99
chocolate, 188
  Chocolate Macaroons, 188
  Mini Chocolate Chunk Banana Sandwiches, 180
  Short-Grain Brown Rice Pudding with Chocolate Wafers (tip), 193
cholesterol, 136, 218
chromium, 50
Chunky Pineapple Ice Pops, 175
cinnamon, 100
  Applesauce, My Mom's, 186
  Nectarine and Orange Compote, 117
Citrus BBQ–Glazed Baby Back Ribs, 232
Citrus Fruit Salad with Fresh Basil, 122
Classic Beef and Barley Stew, 156
coconut. *See also* coconut milk
  Chocolate Macaroons, 188
  Strawberries and Coconut Cream, 184
coconut milk, 123
  Carrot Purée (variation), 44
  Papaya and Coconut Milk Purée, 123
cod, 227
  Butter-Crusted Black Cod with Heirloom Tomatoes, 226
corn. *See also* cornmeal
  Barbecued Corn, Best-Ever, 136
  Corn and Chickpea Chowder, 127
  Cucumber Salad with Smoked Salmon, 210
  Pacific Salmon Cakes, 155
  Veal Rib Chops with Fresh Corn and Asparagus Succotash, 238
cornmeal
  Fennel and Apple–Stuffed Pork Chops, 158

Soft Polenta with Cheddar Cheese and
  Broccoli Florets, 143
couscous, 225
  Israeli Couscous with Black Tiger Shrimp
    and Shrimp "Bisque", 224
  Israeli Couscous with Grated Carrots and
    Chives, 144
cranberries, 19
  Cranberry Phyllo "Pinwheels", 196
  Lamb with Parsnips and Dried Cranberries,
    111
  Roasted Summer Fruit (tip), 120
  Short-Grain Brown Rice Pudding with
    Chocolate Wafers (tip), 193
cream, whipping
  Broccoli, Potato and Spinach Pie, 133
  Celery Root and Chicken Purée (variation),
    72
  Pomegranate and Kiwi Purée with Crème
    Fraîche, 189
  Roasted Summer Fruit Smoothie (tip), 121
  Strawberries and Coconut Cream, 184
Creamy Brown Rice and Fresh Basil, 142
Crispy Potato Galette, 132
cross-contamination, 26–27, 53
cucumber
  Avocado, Carrot and Cucumber Purée, 70
  Barley Salad with Apples and Sugar Snap
    Peas, 215
  Cucumber Salad with Smoked Salmon, 210
cynarin, 125

d

dates, 110
  Applesauce, My Mom's (tip), 186
  Beef Tenderloin and Dates, 110
desserts, 67, 146, 170–71, 173, 180, 183–95
DHA (docosahexanenoic acid), 154
Diced Potato Gratin, 87
dips, 66, 68, 70, 104, 123, 178, 205
dressings. See sauces and dressings
drinks, 37, 69. See also smoothies
duck
  Corn and Chickpea Chowder (variation), 127
  Oven-Roasted Duck Confit with Fresh
    Thyme, 166
  Red Cabbage with Duck Confit, 167

e

eggplant, 86
  Eggplant Parmesan, The Best, 84
  Mediterranean Fried Eggplant, 86
  Ratatouille Vegetables, 101
eggs, 135, 217
  Cheesecake Soufflé, 190
  Chocolate Macaroons, 188
  Egg and Sweet Pepper Fried Rice, 91
  French Toast with Fresh Peaches and Peachy
    Maple Syrup, 148
  Red Potato Salad with Cheddar Cheese and
    Boiled Eggs, 135
  Whole-Grain Oat Crêpes with Warm
    Bananas, 146
enzymes, 69, 90, 187

f

fat, 21, 75, 179. See also omega-3/omega-6
  fatty acids
  essential fatty acids, 21–23
fennel, 158
  Alaskan Halibut en Papillote, 152
  Fennel and Apple–Stuffed Pork Chops,
    158
  Fennel and Orange Sauté, 130
  Red Cabbage, Fennel and Apple Purée,
    96
  White Bean and Fennel Purée, 104
fiber, 41, 194, 237
figs, 56
  Apple and Fig Brown Rice Cereal, 56
  Applesauce, My Mom's (tip), 186
  Berry-Glazed Fig Tart, 194
finger foods, 81, 114
fish and seafood, 22. See also cod; salmon;
  tuna
  Alaskan Halibut en Papillote, 152
  "Fish Sticks", World's Best, 150
  Israeli Couscous with Black Tiger Shrimp
    and Shrimp "Bisque", 224
flavonoids, 87, 89, 173, 197
flours, 51
folate (folic acid), 64, 126, 213
food poisoning, 206
food shopping, 151, 185

French Toast with Fresh Peaches and Peachy
Maple Syrup, 148
Fresh Apricot Purée, 37
Fresh Herb–Crusted Veal Chops, 161
Fresh Soy Bean Hummus, 103
Frozen Blueberry Sorbet, 183
Frozen Fruit Snacks, 173
Frozen Mango Mousse, 187
fructose, 177
fruit, 18, 19, 27, 122, 175. *See also specific*
types of fruit
Frozen Fruit Snacks, 173
Pork with Red Cabbage (tip), 160
Roasted Summer Fruit Smoothie, 121

g

garlic, 88
Basic Sweet-and-Sour Sauce, 209
"Cassoulet" of Black-Eyed Peas, Chorizo
Sausage and NY Steak, 236
Chive Parsley "Pistou", 99
Fresh Soy Bean Hummus, 103
Onion Soup with Cornish Hen, 163
Oven-Roasted Artichokes, 124
Poached Garlic Cloves with Fresh Thyme
and Sour Cream, 88
Potato, Parsnip and Chicken Soup with
Chive Parsley "Pistou", 98
Quick Mushroom Soup, 126
Roasted Cherry Tomato Vinaigrette, 204
Roasted Chicken Stock, 202
Sliced NY Steak with Mushroom Duxelles
and Fresh Horseradish, 240
Veal Rib Chops with Fresh Corn and
Asparagus Succotash, 238
Vegetable Stock, 201
Whole Roasted Chicken Stuffed with Lime
and Green Onions (tip), 230
gingerroot, 92
Bok Choy with Fresh Ginger, 92
Carrot Purée (variation), 44
Egg and Sweet Pepper Fried Rice, 91
Papaya and Coconut Milk Purée, 123
glycemic index, 138
grains, 24, 27, 50
whole, 24, 55, 147, 172
Gramma Jean's Turkey Meatloaf, 164

grapefruit and grapefruit juice
Applesauce, My Mom's, 186
Citrus Fruit Salad with Fresh Basil, 122
grapes
Frozen Fruit Snacks, 173
Whole-Grain Oat Cereal with Grapes, 53
Green Bean Purée with Fresh Basil, 61
greens, salad
Pacific Salmon Cakes (variation), 155
Salmon en Croute with Arugula Salad,
228
Grilled Asparagus with Three Cheeses, 134
Grilled Chicken and Avocado, 75
Grilled Portobello Mushroom Stack with Goat
Cheese, 220
Guacamole, 182

h

herbs, 100. *See also specific herbs*
Fresh Herb–Crusted Veal Chops, 161
Mediterranean Fried Eggplant (tip), 86
Warm Barley with Fresh Herbs and
Parmesan Cheese, 140
honey
Basic Sweet-and-Sour Sauce, 209
Citrus BBQ–Glazed Baby Back Ribs, 232
Honey Mustard–Glazed Salmon with
Avocado, 218
Honeydew, Blueberry and Mint Purée, 62
horseradish, 206, 241
Lemon Horseradish Aioli, 206
Sliced NY Steak with Mushroom Duxelles
and Fresh Horseradish, 240
hyaluronic acid, 122

i

ice cream
Mini Chocolate Chunk Banana Sandwiches
(variation) 3, 180
Roasted Summer Fruit Smoothie (tip), 121
insulin, 134
iron, 23, 24, 33, 57, 129
Israeli Couscous with Black Tiger Shrimp and
Shrimp "Bisque", 224
Israeli Couscous with Grated Carrots and
Chives, 144

j

Jasmine Rice with Butternut Squash and Saffron, 145
Jonah's "Mac and Cheese", 138

k

kiwi, 189
Pomegranate and Kiwi Purée with Crème Fraîche, 189

l

lamb
Lamb with Parsnips and Dried Cranberries, 111
Spice-Rubbed Rack of Lamb, 242
Sweet Peas, Lamb and Parsnip, 73
leeks
Chicken with Roasted Butternut Squash and Leeks, 108
Stewed Leeks with Butter, 83
Whole Roasted Chicken Stuffed with Lime and Green Onions (tip), 230
legumes, 105, 237. See also beans; chickpeas; peas, dried
lemon, 207
Caper and Lemon Remoulade, 207
Chickpea, Grape Tomato and Feta Salad, 212
Citrus BBQ–Glazed Baby Back Ribs, 232
Lemon Horseradish Aioli, 206
Poached Whole Artichokes with Lemon Horseradish Aioli, 216
lentils
Chicken and Red Lentils, 74
Red Lentil and Apple, 71
limonoids, 207
linoleic acid, 23
lycopene, 94, 204

m

"Mac and Cheese", Jonah's, 138
magnesium, 153
manganese, 192

mango, 39, 187
Frozen Mango Mousse, 187
Mango Purée, 39
maple syrup, 149, 192
Citrus Fruit Salad with Fresh Basil, 122
Cranberry Phyllo "Pinwheels", 196
French Toast with Fresh Peaches and Peachy Maple Syrup, 148
Maple Syrup–Glazed Pineapple, 192
Mini Sweet Potato Muffins with Maple Syrup Glaze, 176
Pomegranate and Kiwi Purée with Crème Fraîche, 189
Short-Grain Brown Rice Pudding with Chocolate Wafers, 193
Simple Millet Cereal (variation), 49
mayonnaise
Caper and Lemon Remoulade, 207
homemade, 216
Lemon Horseradish Aioli, 206
mealtimes, 16, 118
meat, 19–20, 93, 111, 233, 240. See also specific types of meat
Mediterranean Fried Eggplant, 86
melatonin, 165
melon
Frozen Blueberry Sorbet (variation), 183
Honeydew, Blueberry and Mint Purée, 62
Watermelon, Peach and Blueberry Purée, 69
methionine, 74
milk
Broccoli, Potato and Spinach Pie (tip), 133
Celery Root and Chicken Purée (variation), 72
Cheddar Cheese Dip, 178
Chicken with Roasted Butternut Squash and Leeks (variation), 108
Creamy Brown Rice and Fresh Basil, 142
Diced Potato Gratin, 87
Israeli Couscous with Black Tiger Shrimp and Shrimp "Bisque", 224
Quick Mushroom Soup, 126
Short-Grain Brown Rice Pudding with Chocolate Wafers, 193
Whole-Grain Oat Crêpes with Warm Bananas, 146

millet and millet flour, 49, 51, 90
  Millet and Cauliflower with Fresh Oregano, 141
  Millet Cereal with Crushed Bananas and Sour Cream, 90
  Simple Millet Cereal, 49
Mini Chocolate Chunk Banana Sandwiches, 180
Mini Sweet Potato Muffins with Maple Syrup Glaze, 176
mint, 62
  Avocado, Carrot and Cucumber Purée, 70
  Cauliflower and Chickpea Chowder, 66
  Honeydew, Blueberry and Mint Purée, 62
  Roasted Summer Fruit Smoothie, 121
  Sweet Pea Purée (variation), 45
muffins, 176
mushrooms, 126
  Grilled Portobello Mushroom Stack with Goat Cheese, 220
  Quick Mushroom Soup, 126
  Salmon en Croute with Arugula Salad, 228
  Sliced NY Steak with Mushroom Duxelles and Fresh Horseradish, 240
  Turkey Meatloaf, Gramma Jean's, 164
mustard
  Honey Mustard–Glazed Salmon with Avocado, 218
  Sliced NY Steak with Mushroom Duxelles and Fresh Horseradish, 240
My Mom's Applesauce, 186

n
nectarines
  Applesauce, My Mom's, 186
  Nectarine and Carrot Purée, 59
  Nectarine and Orange Compote, 117
noodles and pasta
  "Mac and Cheese", Jonah's, 138
  Oven-Roasted Red Peppers (variation), 208
  Sweet Potato Purée (variation), 41
nutrients, 15, 19, 20–21, 71. See also specific nutrients
nuts and seeds, 22
  Chive Parsley "Pistou" (tip), 99
  Honey Mustard–Glazed Salmon with Avocado, 218

Poppy Seed–Crusted Yellowfin Tuna with Roasted Shallots, 222

O
oats and oat flour, 51, 53
  Cranberry Phyllo "Pinwheels", 196
  Whole-Grain Oat Cereal with Grapes, 53
  Whole-Grain Oat Crêpes with Warm Bananas, 146
oils, 131, 144
omega-3 fatty acids, 21–22, 153, 155, 179
omega-6 fatty acids, 23, 179, 211
onions
  Basic Sweet-and-Sour Sauce, 209
  Chickpea, Grape Tomato and Feta Salad, 212
  Citrus BBQ–Glazed Baby Back Ribs, 232
  Egg and Sweet Pepper Fried Rice, 91
  Onion Soup with Cornish Hen, 163
  Pacific Salmon Cakes, 155
  Pork Tenderloin and Peaches, 109
  Quick Mushroom Soup, 126
  Ratatouille Vegetables, 101
  Roasted Chicken Stock, 202
  Roasted Onion Soubise, 97
  Sautéed Chard with Apples, 102
  Soft Polenta with Cheddar Cheese and Broccoli Florets (variation), 143
  Vegetable Stock, 201
  Whole Roasted Chicken Stuffed with Lime and Green Onions, 230
oranges and orange juice, 130
  Barley Salad with Apples and Sugar Snap Peas, 215
  Citrus BBQ–Glazed Baby Back Ribs, 232
  Citrus Fruit Salad with Fresh Basil, 122
  Fennel and Orange Sauté, 130
  Honeydew, Blueberry and Mint Purée (variation), 62
  Nectarine and Orange Compote, 117
  Watermelon, Peach and Blueberry Purée (variation), 69
oregano, 141
  Millet and Cauliflower with Fresh Oregano, 141
organic foods, 16–20

Oven-Roasted Artichokes, 124
Oven-Roasted Cauliflower with Fresh Herbs, 137
Oven-Roasted Cherry Tomato Purée, 94
Oven-Roasted Chicken with Dried Apricots, 106
Oven-Roasted Cornish Hen with Sage, 234
Oven-Roasted Duck Confit with Fresh Thyme, 166
Oven-Roasted Red Peppers, 208

p

Pacific Salmon Cakes, 155
Papaya and Coconut Milk Purée, 123
parsley
    Butter-Crusted Black Cod with Heirloom Tomatoes, 226
    Chive Parsley "Pistou", 99
    Oven-Roasted Cauliflower with Fresh Herbs, 137
    Roasted Chicken Stock, 202
parsnips, 47
    Basic Sweet-and-Sour Sauce, 209
    Caramelized Parsnip Purée, 47
    "Cassoulet" of Black-Eyed Peas, Chorizo Sausage and NY Steak, 236
    Cauliflower and Parsnip Purée, 65
    Lamb with Parsnips and Dried Cranberries, 111
    Potato, Parsnip and Chicken Soup with Chive Parsley "Pistou", 98
    Roasted Chicken Stock, 202
    Sweet Peas, Lamb and Parsnip, 73
    Turnip and Parsnip "Smash", 95
    Vegetable Stock, 201
pasta. See noodles and pasta
pastry
    Berry-Glazed Fig Tart, 194
    Cranberry Phyllo "Pinwheels", 196
    Salmon en Croute with Arugula Salad, 228
peaches
    French Toast with Fresh Peaches and Peachy Maple Syrup, 148
    Nectarine and Carrot Purée (tip), 59
    Pork Tenderloin and Peaches, 109
    Roasted Summer Fruit, 120
    Watermelon, Peach and Blueberry Purée, 69

pears, 36
    Bosc Pear Purée, 36
    Roasted Apple, Blueberry and Pear, 58
    Tofu, Bosc Pears and Banana, 57
peas, dried
    Carrot and Split Pea Purée, 68
    "Cassoulet" of Black-Eyed Peas, Chorizo Sausage and NY Steak, 236
peas, green, 45, 215
    Barley Salad with Apples and Sugar Snap Peas, 215
    Sweet Pea Purée, 45
    Sweet Peas, Lamb and Parsnip, 73
pesticides, 16–19
phenylalanine, 74
phosphorus, 72
pineapple, 119
    Chunky Pineapple Ice Pops, 175
    Maple Syrup–Glazed Pineapple, 192
    Warm Pineapple with Cottage Cheese and Basil, 119
pizza, 83
plums, 174
    Applesauce, My Mom's (tip), 186
    "Chips and Salsa" — Parmesan Cheese Crisps with Plum Salsa, 174
    Plum and Blueberry Purée, 63
    Roasted Summer Fruit, 120
Poached Garlic Cloves with Fresh Thyme and Sour Cream, 88
Poached Whole Artichokes with Lemon Horseradish Aioli, 216
Pomegranate and Kiwi Purée with Crème Fraîche, 189
Poppy Seed–Crusted Yellowfin Tuna with Roasted Shallots, 222
pork. See also bacon
    Citrus BBQ–Glazed Baby Back Ribs, 232
    Fennel and Apple–Stuffed Pork Chops, 158
    Pork Tenderloin and Peaches, 109
    Pork with Red Cabbage, 160
potassium, 128
potatoes, 87, 132. See also sweet potatoes
    Broccoli, Potato and Spinach Pie, 133
    Crispy Potato Galette, 132
    Diced Potato Gratin, 87
    Green Bean Purée with Fresh Basil (variation), 61

potatoes (*continued*)
  Potato, Parsnip and Chicken Soup with
    Chive Parsley "Pistou", 98
  Red Potato Salad with Cheddar Cheese and
    Boiled Eggs, 135
  Salmon, Potato and Cauliflower, 154
  "Smashed" Baby Potatoes, 131
poultry, 19–20, 107, 231. *See also* chicken;
    duck; turkey
  Onion Soup with Cornish Hen, 163
  Oven-Roasted Cornish Hen with Sage,
    234
prebiotics, 97
proanthocyanidins, 63
probiotics, 82
protein sources, 121, 129
prunes, 174
purées, 24–47, 57–76, 94, 96, 104, 123

q

quercetin, 19, 197
Quick Mushroom Soup, 126
quinoa, 48
  Basic Quinoa, 48
  Quinoa and Banana Purée, 54
  Summer Cherry and Quinoa, 89

r

raspberries
  Roasted Summer Fruit, 120
  Strawberries with Granny Smith Apples
    (tip), 116
Ratatouille Vegetables, 101
raw foods, 20–21
Red Cabbage, Fennel and Apple Purée, 96
Red Cabbage with Duck Confit, 167
Red Lentil and Apple, 71
Red Potato Salad with Cheddar Cheese and
    Boiled Eggs, 135
resveratrol, 173
rice, 142, 193. *See also* rice flour
  Creamy Brown Rice and Fresh Basil,
    142
  Egg and Sweet Pepper Fried Rice, 91
  Jasmine Rice with Butternut Squash and
    Saffron, 145

Short-Grain Brown Rice Pudding with
    Chocolate Wafers, 193
rice flour, 51
  Apple and Fig Brown Rice Cereal, 56
  Brown Rice Cereal, 50
  Roasted Apple, Blueberry and Pear, 58
  Roasted Banana Purée, 34
  Roasted Beet Purée, 46
  Roasted Beet Salad, 214
  Roasted Cherry Tomato Vinaigrette, 204
  Roasted Chicken Stock, 202
  Roasted Onion Soubise, 97
  Roasted Red Pepper Vinaigrette, 205
  Roasted Summer Fruit, 120
  Roasted Summer Fruit Smoothie, 121
  Roasted Sweet Potato Purée, 42

s

saffron, 145
  Jasmine Rice with Butternut Squash and
    Saffron, 145
sage, 234
  Oven-Roasted Cornish Hen with Sage, 234
  Quick Mushroom Soup, 126
salads, 48, 76, 122, 132, 210–15
salmon, 155, 211
  Crispy Potato Galette (variation), 132
  Cucumber Salad with Smoked Salmon, 210
  Honey Mustard–Glazed Salmon with
    Avocado, 218
  Pacific Salmon Cakes, 155
  Salmon, Potato and Cauliflower, 154
  Salmon en Croute with Arugula Salad, 228
salt, 150, 238
sandwiches and wraps, 74, 75
saturated fat, 75, 179
sauces and dressings, 46, 72, 97, 110, 204–9
Sautéed Chard with Apples, 102
seaweed, 105
selenium, 193
serotonin, 165
Short-Grain Brown Rice Pudding with
    Chocolate Wafers, 193
Simple Barley Cereal, 52
Simple Millet Cereal, 49
Sliced NY Steak with Mushroom Duxelles
    and Fresh Horseradish, 240

"Smashed" Baby Potatoes, 131
smoothies, 39, 58, 121
snacks, 59, 115, 170, 172–82
sodium, 105
Soft Polenta with Cheddar Cheese and Broccoli
    Florets, 143
soups and stocks, 44, 62, 66, 98, 126–28,
    163, 201–2
sour cream
    Cauliflower and Chickpea Chowder
        (variation), 66
    Cheddar Cheese Dip, 178
    Cranberry Phyllo "Pinwheels", 196
    "Mac and Cheese", Jonah's, 138
    Millet Cereal with Crushed Bananas and
        Sour Cream, 90
    Poached Garlic Cloves with Fresh Thyme
        and Sour Cream, 88
    Pomegranate and Kiwi Purée with Crème
        Fraîche (tip), 189
    Roasted Summer Fruit Smoothie (tip), 121
    Sour Cream "Latkes", 172
    Turnip and Parsnip "Smash" (variation), 95
soy, 21, 103
    Fresh Soy Bean Hummus, 103
    Tofu, Bosc Pears and Banana, 57
Spice-Rubbed Rack of Lamb, 242
spices, 100, 242, 243
spinach, 133
    Broccoli, Potato and Spinach Pie, 133
    Crispy Potato Galette (variation), 132
spreads, 103, 116
squash, 43
    Acorn Squash Purée, 43
    Apricot Acorn Squash Purée, 60
    Chicken with Roasted Butternut Squash and
        Leeks, 108
    Jasmine Rice with Butternut Squash and
        Saffron, 145
    Roasted Sweet Potato Purée (tip), 42
    Zucchini and Basil Purée (tip), 64
Stewed Leeks with Butter, 83
strawberries, 184, 185
    Apple and Strawberry Compote, 118
    Roasted Summer Fruit, 120
    Strawberries and Coconut Cream, 184
    Strawberries with Granny Smith Apples, 116
sugar, cane, 185

sulforaphane, 85, 137
sulfur, 83
Summer Cherry and Quinoa, 89
Sweet Pea Purée, 45
Sweet Peas, Lamb and Parsnip, 73
sweet potatoes, 41, 42
    "Mac and Cheese", Jonah's, 138
    Mini Sweet Potato Muffins with Maple Syrup
        Glaze, 176
    Roasted Sweet Potato Purée, 42
    Sweet Potato Purée, 41
sweeteners, 171, 185
Swiss chard, 102
    Sautéed Chard with Apples, 102

t

teething pain, 67
thyme, 166
    Butter-Crusted Black Cod with Heirloom
        Tomatoes, 226
    Classic Beef and Barley Stew, 156
    Onion Soup with Cornish Hen, 163
    Oven-Roasted Artichokes, 124
    Oven-Roasted Cauliflower with Fresh Herbs,
        137
    Oven-Roasted Cherry Tomato Purée, 94
    Oven-Roasted Duck Confit with Fresh
        Thyme, 166
    Oven-Roasted Red Peppers, 208
    Poached Garlic Cloves with Fresh Thyme
        and Sour Cream, 88
    Poached Whole Artichokes with Lemon
        Horseradish Aioli, 216
    Poppy Seed–Crusted Yellowfin Tuna with
        Roasted Shallots, 222
    Pork with Red Cabbage, 160
    Ratatouille Vegetables, 101
    Veal Rib Chops with Fresh Corn and
        Asparagus Succotash, 238
Tofu, Bosc Pears and Banana, 57
tomatoes, 204
    Asparagus and Roasted Tomato, 128
    Butter-Crusted Black Cod with Heirloom
        Tomatoes, 226
    Chicken and Red Lentils (variation), 74
    Chickpea, Grape Tomato and Feta Salad,
        212

tomatoes (*continued*)

Eggplant Parmesan, The Best, 84

Grilled Chicken and Avocado (variation), 75

Guacamole, 182

Israeli Couscous with Black Tiger Shrimp and Shrimp "Bisque", 224

Oven-Roasted Cherry Tomato Purée, 94

Papaya and Coconut Milk Purée (tip), 123

Roasted Cherry Tomato Vinaigrette, 204

Zucchini and Basil Purée (variation), 64

trans fats, 179

tryptophan, 165

tuna, 223

Poppy Seed–Crusted Yellowfin Tuna with Roasted Shallots, 222

Ratatouille Vegetables (variation), 101

turkey

Oven-Roasted Artichokes (tip), 124

Turkey Meatloaf, Gramma Jean's, 164

turnips, 95

"Cassoulet" of Black-Eyed Peas, Chorizo Sausage and NY Steak, 236

Turnip and Parsnip "Smash", 95

V

vanilla bean

Mini Sweet Potato Muffins with Maple Syrup Glaze, 176

Vanilla Bean Yogurt, 82

veal, 161

Fresh Herb–Crusted Veal Chops, 161

Veal Rib Chops with Fresh Corn and Asparagus Succotash, 238

vegetables, 18, 19, 20–21, 27, 101. *See also specific vegetables*

Basic Quinoa (variation), 48

Brussels Sprout Gratin (variation), 85

Cheddar Cheese Dip (tip), 178

Vegetable Stock, 201

vegetarianism, 24, 104, 129

vitamin A, 39, 44, 160

vitamin B_3, 109

vitamin B_{12}, 129, 156

vitamin C, 58, 91

vitamin D, 129, 136

vitamin K, 65

W

Warm Barley with Fresh Herbs and Parmesan Cheese, 140

Warm Pineapple with Cottage Cheese and Basil, 119

watermelon

Frozen Blueberry Sorbet (variation), 183

Watermelon, Peach and Blueberry Purée, 69

White Bean and Fennel Purée, 104

White Navy Bean and Beef Tenderloin Purée, 76

Whole-Grain Oat Cereal with Grapes, 53

Whole-Grain Oat Crêpes with Warm Bananas, 146

Whole Roasted Chicken Stuffed with Lime and Green Onions, 230

World's Best "Fish Sticks", 150

Y

yogurt, 82

Carrot and Split Pea Purée (variation), 68

Cheddar Cheese Dip, 178

Cucumber Salad with Smoked Salmon, 210

Nectarine and Carrot Purée (variation), 59

Roasted Apple, Blueberry and Pear (variation), 58

Roasted Summer Fruit Smoothie, 121

Vanilla Bean Yogurt, 82

Z

zinc, 76, 192

zucchini, 64

Ratatouille Vegetables, 101

Zucchini and Basil Purée, 64